# WHEN A LOVED ONE IS DYING

# WHEN A LOVED ONE IS DYING

## Conversations About Care, Connection, and Coping

MAUREEN GRODEN, RN

Johns Hopkins University Press
*Baltimore*

First printed in the United States of America on acid-free paper
9 8 7 6 5 4 3 2 1

Johns Hopkins University Press
2715 North Charles Street
Baltimore, Maryland 21218
www.press.jhu.edu

Library of Congress Cataloging-in-Publication Data

Names: Groden, Maureen, 1955– author
Title: When a loved one is dying : conversations about care, connection, and coping / Maureen Groden, RN.
Description: Baltimore : Johns Hopkins University Press, 2026. | Includes bibliographical references and index.
Identifiers: LCCN 2025024336 | ISBN 9781421453934 hardcover | ISBN 9781421453941 paperback | ISBN 9781421453958 ebook
Subjects: LCSH: Death—Psychological aspects | Terminal care | Grief
Classification: LCC BF789.D4 G757 2026
LC record available at https://lccn.loc.gov/2025024336

A catalog record for this book is available from the British Library.



EU GPSR Authorized Representative
LOGOS EUROPE, 9 rue Nicolas Poussin,
17000, La Rochelle, France
E-mail: Contact@logoseurope.eu

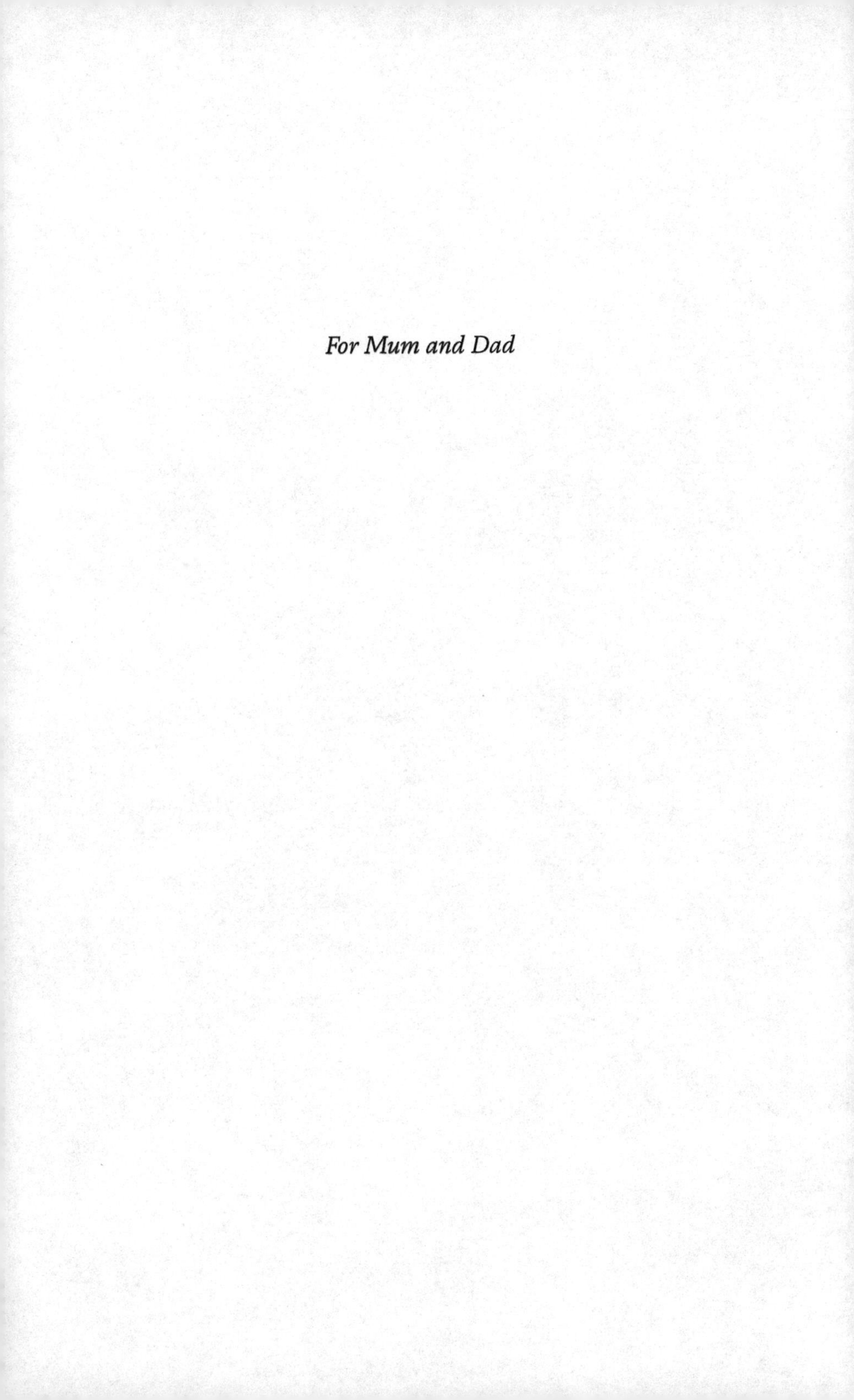

*For Mum and Dad*

# CONTENTS

INTRODUCTION

# Why Talk About Death?

Dealing with an end-of-life disease brings up questions about what treatment to have, whether the treatment is going to work, and at what point people should forgo treatment to focus on living out their lives without a lot of medical tests, treatments, and hospitalizations. Many complex emotions may arise; anxiety, sadness, and fear are commonly felt. People often reflect on their life, relationships, and beliefs about religion, spirituality, and life after death. Philosophical questions also arise, such as the meaning of hope, suffering, and forgiveness. When diseases reach the point of being serious or terminal, they often cause pain, difficulty breathing, fatigue, or other distressing symptoms. How well these are relieved depends on many factors, such as the knowledge and beliefs of individuals and families, and the expertise of health care providers.

With all of these deep human values and experiences, it's not hard to understand why dying, relationships, and death aren't talked about more. It's overwhelming and profoundly sad. However, knowing what questions frequently come up, what often happens during the dying process, and how to care for someone who is dying can help families have a much better experience when the time comes. Additionally, how the experience of dying goes for someone, whether good or bad, can profoundly affect families for the rest of their lives.

I have been a hospice nurse for several decades. Caring for people who are dying has been the privilege of my personal and professional life. Throughout my career, I have been drawn to the study of humanism and the relationships between people when a loved one is at the end of life. What I believe is that every single person in this world is unique. The richness of an individual's history, culture, religion, personality, strength, and resolve will always fascinate me. It has also given me the conviction that patients and their families deserve to be treated with the utmost respect and dignity when they receive health care. What I have learned is that relief of pain and suffering helps people not only have a better quality of life but also a peaceful death.

I wrote this book to help people understand what happens when someone is dying and how to care for them. By sharing stories about families who have faced this end-of-life journey, I hope people can become more familiar and comfortable with dying, death, and hospice care. These stories are meant to illuminate this experience for families, not to replace medical advice provided in specific circumstances. I am grateful for the many people who have opened their hearts and homes to me at such an intimate family time. Their names and scenarios have been changed to protect their privacy.

This book begins with the story of Alice, who abruptly learns that she has a terminal illness. Unfortunately, sometimes as we go about our daily lives, a family illness or death can shock us and change our lives forever. Alice and her family deal with many common experiences that happen when someone is going through the dying process.

The next several chapters tell stories about families who are facing the often confusing decisions about health care treatment, prognosis, and end-of-life care, including the story of my own mother and the experiences our family went through when she got sick, how we dealt with it, and what decisions she and our family made.

Many chapters in the middle of the book are stories about people who are dealing with symptoms and about how their families worked with hospice to manage these difficult experiences. The final chapters share stories about the emotional and spiritual connections that people have and what it means to say goodbye when someone dies. All of the stories end with reflections that I hope will shed light on the care of a loved one who is dying.

These stories may elicit strong memories and emotions. The scenarios and family relationships might impress you as vivid and realistic. It may help to read only a few chapters at a time or to talk with loved ones about the stories and your reactions to them. Take good care as you read through these stories and the reflections that follow.

People who are sick or dying are not any less than who they have ever been. People lose weight, their color changes, and they look very different when they are sick. The dying process, and all the changes that go with it, is a normal and natural process. This certainly doesn't make it any less sad. How people look or how they act in the final days and weeks of their lives doesn't always indicate suffering, however. Perhaps if we talk more about dying and death and become more familiar with this stage of life, we can begin to untangle all the uncertainties, emotions, and complexities that go along with it.

Caring for a loved one who is dying can be one of the most rewarding and exhausting experiences of someone's life. Being that close to the edge of life and death can be profound. Sometimes when it seems like all the news in the world is bad news, I am heartened to walk into the lives of families who are caring for someone who is dying. The love that I see and feel always inspires me. I hope these stories help and inspire you too.

CHAPTER 1

# I Can't Believe This Is Happening

Michelle's mind is racing as she forces herself to speak in a measured voice. "Mom, what exactly did the doctor say?" Her mother, Alice, lives three hours away, but her voice on the phone sounds distant. Not curable? Stage IV? More tests? She can't believe what she is hearing. Michelle becomes mesmerized by a bee on the windshield, flailing its wings against the wipers. In the distance, her daughter's school sits placidly in the afternoon sun. In just a minute, the bell will ring and dozens of children will pour out.

*I can't believe this is happening!*

"Mom, what additional tests do they want to do? Did they say when?"

"They're scheduling me for a scan of my chest next week, honey. They want to see if the cancer has spread to my lungs."

Michelle feels a sudden pang in her chest. "Mom, I'm going to try to go with you. I have to go now; school just got out. I'll call you tonight, love you."

Alice hangs up and says under her breath, "You can't fix everything, sweetheart." Alice will just be relieved to know the extent of things. The worst is not knowing and waiting. Three weeks ago, she saw her doctor because she kept losing weight and felt tired all the time. When her blood tests came back abnormal, they did abdominal scans and saw a mass on her pancreas and liver. She underwent an endoscopy last week, and the results of the biopsy confirmed pancreatic cancer that has spread to her liver. The doctor is recommending additional tests to determine where else the cancer may have spread and, therefore, what treatment options might be available.

*I always thought Tom would go first; he's the one who's had all the medical problems. I guess you just never know.*

Alice and her husband, Tom, live in a beautiful seniors' housing development called Riverview. The spacious town houses each have a garage, backyard, and porch. Alice and Tom were one of the first to move there, so they have an end unit with a side yard in addition to the backyard. They love sitting out on the porch and admiring the large rhododendron bushes and, beyond the border, the river walk with benches. They like to watch the people out for a stroll, and when it's quiet, they see a fair amount of wildlife.

Alice and Tom are both retired from teaching careers. Alice taught fifth grade for thirty-five years at the same elementary school, and Tom initially taught high school history but then switched to teaching civics at the local community college. Downsizing five years ago from the large family home was a difficult step, but now that this is happening, Alice is relieved.

*I can't even imagine living at the Elm Street house or trying to move now.*

Alice has never been one to nap. Even after retirement, she has kept busy doing housework, volunteering at the library, and socializing with her friends at Riverview or with her retired teachers group. The group gets together every Friday for breakfast. They call themselves "the Breakfast Club."

Now Alice feels like she's dragging a ten-pound weight around. Even the slightest activity tires her out and makes her breathless. She often wonders if she missed some signs. Perhaps she's been so busy lately that she just wasn't paying attention to her body. Maybe on some level, she knew something was wrong, but she chose to ignore the signs.

*No, things weren't obvious until recently when the fatigue set in. There's no point in my second-guessing.*

"Alice, do you want some lunch?" Tom calls over to her from the kitchen. Their living room and kitchen area span one big open room. Alice loves the way this room turned out. The mint-colored couch and accent chairs are nicely arranged around the jasmine-and-ivory-colored oriental rug. Three large windows, one on the entrance wall and two on the west side, shower the room with bright sun.

"I should," Alice answers from her spot on the couch, where she's reading.

"What do you want? I'll make you something."

"Oh, I don't know," she ponders. "Nothing appeals to me, to be honest. Maybe I'll have a little yogurt and a piece of toast."

They sit at the small kitchen table and chat about upcoming events at the community room and the latest news about this person or that. Alice feels increasingly separated from these everyday conversations, as there's always a parallel monologue running in her head.

*Will I even be here then? How is Tom going to manage?*

"How is your lunch?" Tom asks.

Alice focuses on Tom with effort. "The toast tastes good, but the yogurt tastes like chalk," she tells him. "I better stick with the blended fruit ones. They're smoother." As Tom is talking about the blueberry and peach flavors on sale at the grocery store, Alice feels a dull pain in her stomach and a tightening sensation in her back. She puts her spoon down, takes a deep breath, and places her hand on her upper stomach. Alice has been trying to push herself to eat more high-protein and high-calorie foods, but this pain is happening more and more when she eats. The doctor gave her some pain pills, but she is reluctant to take them. *It'll pass*, she thinks to herself. "Tom, I'm going to lie down for a bit." Holding onto the furniture, she makes her way back to the couch.

Alice doesn't want everyone making a big fuss over her. Her oldest daughter, Emily, lives on the other side of the country and travels a lot. Michelle comes to visit regularly, but she's still several hours away. Andrew is nearby, but they're all so busy with work, children, coaching, and everything else. Michelle is the one she's worried about. Emily has always ruled with her head, practical and ambitious, whereas Michelle has always ruled with her heart, emotional and vulnerable. *I'm afraid she's going to take this very hard.*

*I'm not even sure I have the energy to deal with all of this.*

Just as Alice feared, the tests show that the cancer is also in her right lung. She is referred to an oncologist. Alice and Tom sit in the exam room while the doctor goes over all the tests, scans, percentages, and scenarios. To Alice, it all sounds bleak. She looks over at Tom, who looks so innocent, like one of her fifth-grade boys who forgot his lunch money. She feels worse for him than for herself.

*I can take this, but I'm not sure if he can. He'll just have to, I guess . . .*

The doctor explains that he can offer her chemotherapy. It might extend her prognosis by a few months, but given her age and the extent of the cancer, even with treatment, her prognosis is likely a year or less. Alice feels numb. She is picturing this entire conversation as if she were looking down on it from above.

*All I really want to do is go home*, she says to herself as pleasantries come out of her mouth.

One by one, she tells her children the bad news. Andy stops over after supper and Alice and Tom relay the news from the oncologist. As Alice gently tells Andy about her decision not to get chemotherapy, she can see the worry in his kind blue eyes. He reaches over and gives her a bear hug. Alice knows that Andy has always been good-natured and handles most things with a sense of humor.

*He also has a busy little family, so I think he'll be okay in the long run*, she reassures herself.

Alice glances at the clock on the stove; it's 8:15 p.m., so it's 5:15 p.m. out west. She calls Emily and reaches her just as she is getting home from work. Alice tells Emily about the doctor's appointment, what the tests revealed, and her decision to just live out her life at home as best she can. Emily asks numerous questions about the scans, tumor markers, and treatment decisions. As Alice suspects, Emily seems satisfied with all the answers she gets. She tells her mom how sorry she is that all of this is happening and she offers to come home anytime if needed. Alice tells her that a nurse from hospice will be coming to visit this Saturday to talk about the program and how things work. Alice agrees to call Emily later that day after the meeting.

Alice closes her eyes and takes a deep breath. Tom walks over behind her and wraps his arms loosely around her shoulders. They both know that the most difficult call is yet to come. Michelle will be calling around 9 p.m. when she gets back from the gym. Alice gets up slowly and winces as she puts her hand onto her left side. She walks carefully toward her bedroom, holding onto the furniture and walls as she goes.

*I have a few minutes. I might as well get washed up and put on my nightgown. I wish I could tell Michelle in person, but it's better to tell her right away than to wait.* Alice feels those weights dragging her down again. Only now, she also feels her heart racing and her hands shaking.

"Hi, honey. How was your workout?"

"Good. I'm getting there. Mom, how are you doing? How'd your appointment go?"

Alice braces herself. "I'm sorry, but it's not the best news, Michelle. The tests show that the cancer has also spread to my right lung. That probably explains why I've felt so winded lately." Alice pauses for a few seconds and waits for Michelle to say something. When there's no response, Alice figures that Michelle is weeping but trying to be silent.

"Michelle?"

"I'm sorry, Mom."

Alice reaches over and grabs a tissue. For the first time since the appointment, she feels scared. Her eyes are burning and she feels on the verge of a flood of tears.

Thankfully, Michelle breaks the silence. "What else did he say?"

Alice clears her throat and begins. "The doctor said that he could offer me a course of chemotherapy. Unfortunately, because it's already spread, it probably wouldn't be able to cure the cancer, but it might just buy me a little more time."

"Like how much time, did he say?"

"Well, probably only about a year. Your father and I talked about it, Michelle. I've decided that it's just too much for me to go through, given the extent of things."

"Are you going to get a second opinion? Wouldn't that be a good idea?"

"Honey, I think the scans are pretty conclusive. Again, it just seems like a lot. I'm already dragging; honestly, I don't think I have the energy for it."

"It just seems like there should be something that would help. Can't they operate and remove the tumor? I don't want you to just give up."

"All the options will probably make me feel worse. I know this is really hard for all of us. Believe me, if I thought that anything would help, I would do it." Alice now feels both physically and emotionally exhausted. It's been a long day, to say the least. "Honey, this Saturday, a hospice nurse is coming to visit to talk about their services. I know you were coming anyway, so I asked her to come around three p.m. I would very much like for you to be here. Okay? Andy also said he can make it. I think it would give all of us a chance to talk things over and ask whatever questions we have."

"Yes, of course I'll be there," Michelle says, sniffling. "I love you, Mom. I'm so sorry."

"Good night, sweetheart. I love you too. I'll call you tomorrow."

Alice wipes her eyes and blows her nose. With a deep sigh, she lies back on her pillow and stretches out her legs. She is so relieved to finally be back in bed. As she drifts off to sleep, Alice remembers all the times when Michelle used to go to sleepovers and summer camps. She would always tell her that if she got scared being away from home, she could just look up to the sky and find the stars and the moon. Alice would reassure her that she didn't need to be afraid. Her mom would also be looking at those same stars and moon. That way she wouldn't be alone.

Saturday afternoon, Michelle bustles in carrying a large bouquet of red, yellow, and purple flowers in one hand and a bag of food in the other. “Hi, Mom and Dad! I brought the makings for some chicken and vegetable soup.” She drops everything on the table and embraces her mom for several minutes, resting her head on her shoulder.

“Thank you so much, sweetheart. We’ll get through this.”

“When’s Andy coming over?” Michelle asks.

“He should be here shortly; he’s coaching a soccer game, but he said he’ll be here around two thirty p.m.”

“Mom, are you ready for this? I mean, will this be hard for you?”

“Honestly, Michelle, I’m better off having the information about what to expect. I think I get more worried and anxious when I don’t know what’s going on.”

“You and me both, Mom.”

Michelle and Tom move around the kitchen chatting about family news and putting the flowers in a vase and the food in the refrigerator. Alice settles into her usual place on the couch.

She closes her eyes and basks in the warm sun that is flooding the living room. Soon Andy arrives. They all catch up while Michelle puts out tea, cider, crackers, and cheese for everyone.

Just as they are settling into the living room with Alice, the doorbell rings. Tom jumps up, answers the door, and welcomes Charlene, the hospice nurse.

“Hi, everyone. I’m Charlene. What a beautiful room this is!”

“Thank you,” Tom says. “We really love it here.”

By now, the afternoon sun has warmed up the room, but it’s almost too bright. Michelle jumps up and lowers the blinds halfway. Tom leads Charlene to the chair next to Alice and they all introduce themselves.

Before beginning the meeting, Charlene asks if Alice is comfortable. After hearing that she is, she asks Alice to tell her a little bit about herself. "You mean my medical condition?" she asks.

"No," Charlene clarifies, "tell me about yourself."

Alice raises her eyebrows and looks up at Charlene; that's not usually how these medical appointments go. Alice tells Charlene about being retired from teaching, how much enjoyment she got from all the students over the years, what she likes to do now, such as reading and listening to opera, who her children and grandchildren are, and how proud she is of all of them.

Charlene then tells her that she is really sorry about the cancer diagnosis and what they all now have to face. She asks Alice about her symptoms, how she is managing, what she is eating, and how she is getting around. Each time she asks Alice a question, Charlene offers advice, such as how to manage the pain, tips on eating, and strategies for conserving energy. Tom and Andy interject additional points or requests for clarification along the way.

Michelle is sitting on the couch next to her mom. Periodically she reaches over and rubs her mom's leg. With tears building up in her eyes, she asks Charlene a number of questions.

"How much of the medicine should she be taking? And should she be going out?"

Charlene calmly explains, "Right now, she has pain medicine that she can take every four hours if she needs it. We pay a lot of attention to managing symptoms, so we'll work with your mom to make sure she's comfortable. And it's fine for her to go out if she feels up to it."

"What should we tell our kids? They're all very close to their Grammy. I don't want to worry them, but they should know."

"Absolutely, Michelle. With kids, it's always best to be honest and to match the information provided with their age. Our hospice team has both social workers and bereavement counselors who help children deal with these situations. We can also help all of you with what to tell them and how to respond to common questions they may ask."

Michelle sits back and cups her tea in both hands.

Charlene turns to Alice. "I want to ask you a question, Alice, that you may or may not be able to answer right now, but perhaps you can think about it. How do you want this to go? In other words, what is most important to you right now?" Charlene asks gently.

Alice answers right away. "I've been thinking about this a lot, ever since the doctor's appointment. Well, I don't want to suffer, and I don't want this to drag on. I don't want Tom and the children to go through that."

"Mom, we don't want you to go through that either!" Michelle adds quickly.

"Yes, I know, Michelle, but . . ." Alice says, trailing off.

Charlene reassures them again that hospice clinicians focus on managing symptoms. "We know how important it is to control pain, nausea, constipation, and any other symptoms that might come up." She reviews Alice's current medication list. Charlene encourages her to take the short-acting pain medicine when the pain first starts. "This type of pain often gets worse, and then it will take longer to control it." She goes on to explain the different types of medicine, what they're used for, and how to take them. Charlene tells them about the services from hospice. We have a team of people who are available to help. "We don't move in, but we are here to help you and your whole family when needed."

Alice decides that this is the type of care that she needs right now. It will also help her family. Later that night, she calls Emily on the phone and tells her about the meeting and relays what Charlene told them about hospice. "Emily, I feel better. I feel like there's a plan."

Over the next two months, Alice is able to get around with a cane. She's only missed one of the Breakfast Club meetings. She finds that if she takes a pain and nausea pill before the breakfast, she does much better. She's had some trouble with constipation, so the doctor started her on a laxative. Besides that, she is doing okay. Tom has surprised her. Besides the shopping, which he usually does anyway, he is doing the laundry and dishes.

*I guess this is just one of the many things to let go of*, she thinks as she closes her eyes and listens to her favorite opera that Andy downloaded onto her phone.

Two weeks later, in the evening, Alice and Tom are in their bedroom. "I think I better call hospice," Tom says to Alice as she rolls over in bed with her head over a basin. Alice nods while holding the wet washcloth on her forehead.

"She was fine until late this afternoon, then she started with some dry heaves. She vomited once, but she really hasn't had much to eat," Tom relays to Olga, the nurse on call. Olga tells him that she will come right over. Alice might need some different medication right now.

It's 9 p.m. when Olga arrives. She enters their large bedroom in the back left corner of the house. Their bed is covered with a beautiful homemade quilt in rich jewel tones. Alice's body looks small in the bed. She is lying on her left side with her left arm over her head and her right arm clutching the basin. Olga asks Alice about how she's feeling, but she can't provide Olga with any details; she just shakes her head. Olga then reviews with Tom what's been going on and what medications she's had. She checks her physical signs and then gives Alice a suppository for the nausea. After calling the hospice doctor on the phone, Olga explains to Alice and Tom the new plan for managing the pain and nausea. "Tonight, you'll start a patch for the pain and a suppository for the nausea. This will allow you to get relief without having to put anything in your stomach for now." Olga confirms that Andy can pick up these medicines at the pharmacy tonight and that Tom is clear on how to administer them. "Please be sure to call me overnight if you don't feel better. Charlene will be back out tomorrow to check on you."

Alice's condition changes rapidly after that night. She is spending most of her time in bed except when she gets up to use the commode. Her skin and eyes have turned a yellowish color and her belly is distended. She's hardly eating anything. Thankfully, she is comfortable. Occasionally, Alice has to take a few drops of the quick-acting pain medicine, but mostly the patch is keeping the pain away.

Michelle takes a family leave from work and stays with her parents for three-to-four-day stretches. She drives home, or her husband and kids visit, at least once a week. Each morning, she gives her mom a sponge bath in bed and then repositions her on her good side for a nap. While her mom is resting, she takes a walk along the river walk and cries. So many questions come to mind, and no answers.

*How am I going to live without her? She is my rock. I'm trying to be strong for Mom and the kids, but I'm a mess. I am so sad, so exhausted. I feel like throwing myself on the ground.*

As she walks by other people on the walk, she straightens up a bit and nods slightly. *Thank goodness for sunglasses!*

As she walks back into the house, it feels like it's wrapped up in warmth, stillness, and sorrow.

During one of the hospice visits, Tom asks Charlene if she would please call Emily to update her on how things are going. "She called last night and is worried about whether she should come or not," Tom tells her.

Charlene calls Emily and gives her a report on how her mother is doing. After updating her on the medical situation, she gently tells Emily, "It's hard to know for sure, but it's likely that your mom is in the final week or two of life. Emily, if it's important for you to see your mom before she dies, then you should come now." For a few seconds, it's quiet. Emily then thanks Charlene and tells her that she will go ahead and make travel arrangements and call her dad.

Over the next week, Alice is no longer eating or drinking anything and is no longer conscious. The priest comes over and gives her the Sacrament of the Anointing of the Sick. Emily and Michelle are now staying overnight and Andy comes over every day. They take turns bathing, changing, and turning their mom. They talk to her about what they are about to do; they reassure her that they will be okay and will take care of Dad. Charlene set up a medication chart and they each write down the medicine names and when they were administered. They play her favorite opera music quietly and they keep a candle burning on her bedside table. It's very peaceful.

One early afternoon, Michelle and Emily are finishing up bathing their mom. They put a pillow under her arms and under her lower legs. They pull up the sheet and blanket to cover her. "Be sure to fold the sheet over the blanket," Emily tells Michelle, as her mother always did. They both smile. "Always the teacher." They empty the wash basin, roll up the laundry, and join Andy and their dad in the kitchen.

"It's so nice to have you kids around again," Tom says. "It's just too bad that it's because of this."

"I know," Emily says.

Michelle tries to make sense of all the emotions she's feeling and the thoughts running through her head.

*How are we going to be as a family without Mom? Whenever Emily or Andy used to tease me, Mom would come to my defense. Now what?*

Her dad continues, "You know, I was thinking back to that first conversation when your mother told Charlene what mattered most to her. Other than a few bad days, I think she's been mostly comfortable. And once things got bad, they happened fast. Thank God for that."

Emily and Tom continue chatting while they put together a spread for lunch with all the food offerings that have filled the refrigerator. Andy's on the phone with his wife, updating her on things. Michelle peeks in at her mom and sees her chest rise slightly.

Over lunch, they talk about who's stopped by, what they've brought, and how their former neighbors and friends are doing. They retell familiar stories about when they were teenagers and the shenanigans they got themselves into. Andy and Michelle give updates on their kids' activities. For a brief moment, life feels normal.

Michelle gets up and tiptoes into the bedroom to check on her mom. The room sounds eerily quiet. The shades are pulled down so all she can see is the silhouette of her mom in the bed. Michelle walks up to the side of the bed and tentatively places her hand on her shoulder. Her eyes widen and she begins to tremble. "Oh no! Mom?!"

Her siblings and dad rush into the room. They all realize that she has just died. Michelle sits on the bed and begins to sob. Emily wraps her arms around her shaking shoulders to comfort her.

Andy stands at the end of the bed, places his hand on the comforter over her toes, and says, "We love you, Mom."

Tom stands opposite Michelle and Emily as tears well up in his eyes. He bends over and kisses Alice on the forehead. "Goodbye, sweetheart."

## REFLECTIONS ON ALICE AND FAMILY

Life takes a number of unexpected turns along the way. Sickness and death often happen at unpredictable times. As with Alice, all of a sudden a loved one could be diagnosed with a terminal illness. Families experience shock and disbelief. Why is this happening? Why her? There is so much fear, worry, and sadness to deal with. Even when people are on hospice and death is expected, it can come as a surprise when it actually happens. I see how often life can change with a phone call or in a heartbeat. It makes me appreciate life. It also makes me grateful for my loved ones and the time I have to spend with them.

There are many questions and concerns that come up regarding medicines at the end of life. Several chapter reflections will address many of these. It's not uncommon, like with Alice, to need changes in medications because of new symptoms or an inability to swallow pills.[1] Managing distressing symptoms is crucial to helping your loved one have a peaceful death.[2]

Whether you are living far away or nearby, it's hard to know when to come to someone's bedside when they're dying. There is no guarantee that you will be present the moment your loved one dies. I am often asked by family members, like Emily, "Should I come now?" She wants to come before her mom dies and stay for the services, but she can't be away for too long. There are often signs that someone is in the final days of life, but it's not always clear.[3] Sometimes, people wait to die until their loved ones arrive. Other times, people die before a family member gets there. Also, many people die when family members leave the room. I don't know why it happens, but it happens frequently. Perhaps they've just been cleaned and resettled, or it might be about privacy. I have found that dying is like going to sleep. If you're comfortable and relaxed, you will drift right off to sleep. But if you're in pain or worried, you can't sleep. Some families hold a vigil for hours at the bedside.[4] They only leave briefly, and that's when their loved one dies. They may hold on to so much regret about leaving the bedside.[5] I think we live with a lot of uncertainty. There are many predictable things that happen when someone is dying, but I think the exact time in which someone naturally leaves this world is a bit of a mystery.

CHAPTER 2

# Does Palliative Care Mean That Mom Is Dying?

Susan quickly takes off her hairnet and washes her hands in the big metal industrial sink in the school cafeteria's kitchen. She grabs her pocketbook from the rusty blue locker and rushes out the door, yelling back to the two other cafeteria workers, "See you tomorrow!"

In unison, they both yell back, "Good luck with your mom!"

Before she drives the ten-minute commute to the hospital, Susan quickly pulls down the visor, slides open the mirror, and reaches up with both hands to fluff up her hair. Her hands are shaking as she reaches into her pocketbook and grabs her lipstick. She steadies her hand and applies lipstick to her upper and lower lips and then presses them together.

Susan has almost come to expect a call from the hospital every month or so. Six times in the last nine months, her mom has been admitted for difficulty breathing because of her heart condition. This time is different, though. The emergency room doctor made a referral for palliative care. Susan remembers feeling a pang in her chest when the doctor suggested that. "She's not ready to die!" she remembers telling him. But he reassured her and her family members that palliative care is not the same as hospice. They will help her mom decide what kind of care she wants and hopefully reduce the number of times she ends up in the hospital. Susan isn't sure what this is all about, but she and her mother and her sister, Janey, are meeting shortly with a doctor and a social worker in the family conference room at the hospital.

Since her mother, Dottie, assigned her as her health care proxy, Susan gets calls all the time from the hospital, doctors, pharmacists, and her sister, Janey. It makes sense; she is the oldest and the most capable, and she lives only a mile away. Sometimes, though, it feels like too much. She worries that she doesn't spend enough time with her husband at her own house.

*I feel spread so thin.*

Even though Janey lives with their mom, she has a mild, and somewhat vague, cognitive disability and relies on Susan to communicate with everyone and organize most of the care. She is grateful, however, that Janey is very devoted to their mom's day-to-day care. Susan is relieved that her mom is not alone and that she and Janey can look after each other. She worries about what will happen when her mom dies; will Janey be able to live on her own?

Dottie was diagnosed with congestive heart failure about ten years ago. She is taking several medicines to strengthen her heart and reduce the fluid buildup in her feet and lungs caused by her weakened heart. Occasionally, she forgets to take her water pill, or she doesn't want to take it because it makes her pee too much. One time, she ran out of medication and Janey forgot to tell Susan to pick up the refill from the pharmacy. Every time she forgets to take her medication, or skips them, her lungs fill up with fluid and she has a hard time breathing. Janey then calls 911 and Dottie goes to the hospital. That's what happened this time too.

When Susan arrives at the hospital, her mom and sister are already sitting in the family room. She immediately notices that her mom's color looks better; she's more pink and less pale than yesterday. She's also breathing easier. Her oxygen tube is positioned in her nose and is attached to a portable tank on the back of her wheelchair. "Hi, Mom, how are you feeling?"

Dottie immediately responds, "Much better! I hope they tell me I can go home!"

Janey is sitting on one end of a blue vinyl couch. Her knees are together and her hands are folded neatly on top of her pocketbook on her lap. "What do they want to talk to us about, Susie?"

Just then, two people come into the family conference room and introduce themselves as Dr. Jeff, a palliative care doctor, and Mary, a social worker. Dr. Jeff has silver hair and a warm, engaging smile. Susan notices that he isn't wearing a white coat. He has a loose plaid shirt on with his name badge clipped to the pocket. After a round of introductions, he sits down in a chair in front of Dottie and explains, "Mary and I are here to talk with you about your illness and how you are all managing. Before we start, though, are you comfortable, Dottie?"

"As much as can be expected," Dottie says, "but I want to go home."

"We're going to help you with that, Dottie," Mary tells them. "But first we want to talk with you about your care and what you'll need at home." Mary leans forward in her chair and looks at Dottie and then at Susan and Janey, both sitting on the couch. Susan's eyes are drawn to Mary's bright turquoise blouse and long colorful skirt. She is holding a pen in her hand and a yellow folder on her lap.

Dr. Jeff starts by asking Dottie a number of questions. "All things considered, Dottie, what's most important to you right now?"

"Well, for one thing, to go home and stay out of the hospital!" Dottie exclaims. "I also haven't been able to get out to church since the last time I was in the hospital three weeks ago. The minister visited me last week, but it's not the same as seeing everyone in church."

"I've been afraid it's too much for you, Mom," Susan interjects. "Your breathing has been too hard." Susan looks over at Janey for agreement. She nods slightly then darts a glance at her mom.

Dottie's daughters tell Dr. Jeff and Mary that it's scary when their mom can't breathe. They don't know what else to do. Susan looks over at her mom. She is tiny, barely 4 feet, 10 inches tall. Her legs are pale and swollen, and her feet barely reach the footrests. She has white hair with loose curls and thick, gold-rimmed glasses that make her eyes look large and bright. Her mom has always been small but mighty. She has firm opinions and convictions and will often share them by extending her arms downward with clenched fists. She does that now and proclaims, "I don't want to live like this!"

"We hear you, Dottie," Mary reassures her. "That's exactly why we want to talk with you and your family about a different approach to your care."

Over the next half hour, Dr. Jeff and Mary ask Dottie several questions about her medical history, day-to-day routine, what she enjoys best, and what makes things difficult.

"I like sitting out on the porch when I feel up to it. I also like cooking and making dinner for Janey and me. Sometimes my legs give out, though, and I have to sit down and catch my breath. Janey and I then watch our shows, *Wheel of Fortune* and *Jeopardy!*."

Susan looks back and forth between Dr. Jeff, Mary, and her mom. She knows that Janey isn't comfortable speaking up in situations like this. Susan fills in the blanks in the conversation when it seems like her mom is going off track, or if she forgets to add an important detail to the story. Susan feels like an interpreter. She tries to capture who her mom is and what matters to her and to also respond to medical questions about her lifestyle and how she manages her illness.

Dr. Jeff and Mary teach Dottie and her daughters about congestive heart failure and the medications. They review ways to prevent and manage fatigue and difficulty breathing. They discuss what Dottie would want for emergency care in the event her heart or lungs stopped working. Dr. Jeff reviews the POLST (Portable Orders for Life Sustaining Treatment) form with them, where it spells out what treatments Dottie would want, such as intravenous fluids, resuscitation, and a breathing tube. In her usual declarative stance, Dottie proclaims, "Not that breathing tube! I had that once—never again!" The doctor reassures Dottie that her treatment choices are documented on the form and he encourages her to put the form on her refrigerator when she gets home.

Mary makes sure that Susan, as the health care proxy, and Janey understand what their mom is deciding. Susan assures them that she does. "Last year, Mom was in the intensive care unit on a respirator. We didn't think she was going to make it. She made us promise that we wouldn't let them put that tube back down her throat. This is really the first time we've talked about it since it happened; I'm glad it's on her record." Susan glances sideways at Janey, whose eyes look watery. She reaches over and gently taps her arm. "That was really scary for all of us."

"So, can I go home now?" Dottie asks them as she glances at both of her daughters.

"Yes, we're going to set up everything you'll need for follow-up care and discharge you tomorrow if all goes well. We'd also like to make a referral for the Palliative Care Home Team to visit you. They will arrange for a visiting nurse and social worker to see you, as well as some rehab to help you get stronger and help you manage your personal care needs. The hope is that with attention to preventing and managing your heart condition and breathing troubles, you will be able to do what you want to do and stay out of the hospital. How does that sound?"

"It sounds like a plan," Susan tells them as she looks to her mom and sister for agreement. As the meeting comes to a close, they say their goodbyes. Janey wheels her mom back toward her hospital room. Susan takes the folder from Mary and continues the conversation, providing them with details about her mom's supply of medication and equipment.

"It feels like a weight has been lifted," Susan tells them. "It was good to get these things out in the open. It went better than I expected."

The following day, Susan makes arrangements to work a half day so she can meet the nurse and social worker at her mom's house by 2 p.m. She knows the routine by now; it usually takes at least an hour to sign all the discharge paperwork and pick up the medicines at the pharmacy. She knows her mom is anxious to get home.

Dottie has lived in her current home for forty-five years. Her husband used to take care of the maintenance, but he died almost fifteen years ago. Now the house is looking old and dilapidated. It is a white two-story clapboard home with a front and back porch. The front porch is in disrepair and boarded up. Everyone enters the home through the cluttered back porch.

Inside, Dottie and Janey live in the four downstairs rooms: the kitchen; the living room, which also serves as Dottie's bedroom; the dining room, which is now Janey's bedroom; and the bathroom. Susan wishes she had more time and money to fix things around there, but she just can't. She has her own house, which currently needs a new roof. Her mom and Janey can't afford to fix it either. Medicines, copays, food, and household items pretty much take up her mom's entire social security check and Janey's disability income.

Susan and Janey meet the ambulance at the house. Dottie knows all the paramedics, and they all know her. They bring her in through the back porch and settle her in the kitchen. The table is full with piles of paper, clothes, bedding, and medical supplies. They add the plastic bags of clothing and medical supplies from the hospital to the pile. Susan looks through all the discharge paperwork and grabs the bright pink POLST form and puts it on the refrigerator. "Mom, this is the form that Dr. Jeff went over with us yesterday; it has to stay on the fridge."

The paramedic is switching the oxygen tubing onto her mom's large tank and turns it on. It makes a loud, familiar beep. "Yes," he agrees. "We look for that form to know what to do if there's an emergency."

"Don't worry. It's going to stay right there!" Dottie reassures them. "Listen, honey, when you go to the store, please get me some more tissues. I'm on my last box."

Susan grabs the folder with the discharge information and her pocketbook. "I will," she says as she heads out the back door.

*Some things seem the same, but some things feel different this time.*

Susan gets back to the house in time to meet with the palliative care nurse, Logan, and the social worker, Amy. She worries that her mom has had a long day and won't be able to participate much in the visit. How wrong she is! When she enters the kitchen, her mom is holding court, telling Logan and Amy her life story. Janey is at the sink, peeling carrots and laughing along with them.

"Welcome home, Dottie," Logan says as he reaches over and gently touches her shoulder. "You must be so glad to be back home."

"You have no idea!" Dottie exclaims as they all settle into chairs and begin the visit.

Amy tells them that she and Logan have received the report from the palliative care meeting at the hospital. They are aware of what decisions were made and what is important to Dottie. "I see that you have signed the POLST form and it's on the refrigerator. I also understand that you do not want resuscitation or a breathing tube, and your hope is to not go back to the hospital, unless you have to for comfort. Is that right, Dottie?"

"That's right!" Dottie says as she nods vigorously. "I've been in the hospital so many times lately, I can't even keep track."

Logan smiles and reassures her that they will help her and her family set up a plan to manage her heart condition and prevent breathing problems. "Our Palliative Care Home Team cares for people who have a serious illness but aren't necessarily in the final months of life. People often continue to get curative medical treatment and even hospitalization, if it's needed," he explains. "We keep a closer eye on you, Dottie, and help you and your family manage at home here."

"Well, that all sounds good, especially if it means not having to go back to the hospital!"

"That would definitely help all of us," Susan agrees.

Logan reaches into his bag and takes out his medical supplies. As he checks Dottie's vital signs, he talks with them about the importance of checking her weight daily, conserving her energy, and managing urination and hygiene, especially with the water pills. He reviews the new orders for the medications and explains how and when to use the oxygen. "Dottie, I am going to write down a step-by-step plan for what you and your daughters should do if you begin to feel short of breath." He opens the bag with the medicine and carefully reviews the labels. He then prefills the liquid medicine in a series of special medicine cups.

Logan tears out a piece of paper from a notebook and writes in large, clear letters:

IF YOU START TO HAVE DIFFICULTY BREATHING, STOP!

SIT DOWN AND PUT YOUR OXYGEN MASK ON.

TAKE THE EMERGENCY MEDICINE FROM THE CUP.

BREATHE IN YOUR NOSE, OUT YOUR MOUTH, AND COUNT TO TEN.

CALL 911 IF YOU STILL CAN'T CATCH YOUR BREATH.

CALL SUSAN AND YOUR DOCTOR.

Logan makes sure that everyone is following along with him as he reviews the plan. "Okay, let's practice these steps while we are all here," he suggests. "Susan, let's have your mom and Janey do this, since you might not be here."

Janey swings around with her eyes wide and says, "But what if it doesn't help?"

Susan reassures Janey that these emergency steps are what their mom wants. "If it will help to keep her home, then it's worth it."

"Janey, honey, I can do this myself!" her mom says. "I just need you to help me like you usually do."

Logan smiles and then guides Dottie and Janey through the steps. Dottie reads each step aloud as she directs Janey on what to do. Janey fumbles with the oxygen tubing as she switches the nose piece over to the mask. Even though she has done this dozens of times, she's never had an audience and now feels like she has to pass a test. Dottie starts to instruct, "Just twist the tube near the blue—"

"I know, I know," Janey interrupts. "It's just that the tubes are getting tangled."

Logan reassures them all that they know what to do; they just need to stay calm and follow the plan. "If this doesn't help your breathing, then you should call the ambulance, but these steps might be enough to prevent another hospitalization."

Logan asks Dottie if she thinks a wheelchair might help her get around and also conserve her energy. After initially declining, she accepts the offer. "I guess I can just put it out on the porch if I don't need it. Besides, it might help me to get out to church one of these weekends."

Logan packs up his medical supplies, reminds Dottie to make sure she takes all of her medicine and weighs herself in the morning, and then makes arrangements to visit the following day.

Amy stays seated at the kitchen table. "If it's okay with you, I'm going to talk with you all a bit more about how you're all managing and what else we could do to help." Amy has noticed that their living space has not had any maintenance done on it for some time. Linoleum patches on the kitchen floor are torn and missing, and paint is cracked and peeling on the wall behind the stove. She worries about their safety and risk for falls. "We work with an elder service agency, River Valley Elder Care, that provides a lot of household chores, meals-on-wheels, and shopping help. Would you want any of these?"

Dottie, Susan, and Janey go back and forth with Amy, telling her what services she has had, what has helped, and what she didn't particularly like. Amy smiles as Dottie makes it crystal clear what kind of help she wants. Amy calls River Valley Elder Care and makes arrangements for someone to come and help clean Dottie's home twice a week and deliver meals at lunchtime. They also have a chore service that will evaluate whether they can help with home repairs and seasonal needs. Amy also reminds them that an occupational therapist and home health aide will visit Dottie and help her manage her day-to-day personal needs. "Until you get stronger, let the aide help you wash up and put your stockings on; that will help Janey too!"

Amy spends a little more time talking with Dottie and her daughters, validating how difficult life has been for them all, particularly over the past two years. "Serious illnesses, like heart disease, can cause a lot of uncertainty. I know it's scary to feel sick and worry about whether you're going to get better or not. It's hard for your daughters too, to see you struggle and also to divide up the help you need. This is normal and common. I will help you work it out, if that will be helpful. They all agreed it would. Susan glances at her mom and then at Janey.

*I don't think we have ever had such a heart-to-heart talk like we've had these last two days. Up until now, we've just reacted to everything.*

As the light shifts in the kitchen to grayish shadows, Amy notices that Dottie's eyelids are heavy and her cheeks are starting to droop. "Well, I think we have covered enough ground for today; is there anything else you can think of?"

"I'll put a call over to the church tomorrow, Mom, and see if Reverend Angie can visit you later this week."

"Tell her to come sometime in the morning. I don't want her coming during my nap time!"

Susan and Amy share a glance and a smile. The woman knows what she wants.

Over the next few weeks, Dottie and Janey have a number of people and services come to their home. They write everything on a calendar to keep it all straight. "I told you we are going to keep a close eye on you!" Logan reminded them at one of his visits.

One afternoon, Dottie just can't catch her breath. Her breathing is deep and crackly. She and Janey follow all of the steps on the note on the fridge. By the time Susan comes over, Dottie is breathing a little easier and directing them both on what to do. Dottie's doctor orders an increase in her water pill for three days, and between the emergency medicines and the new orders, Dottie feels better and is able to stay out of the hospital.

Over the next several months, Dottie holds her own and sticks to her routine. She's even been able to sit out back on the porch several afternoons. She has a few more emergencies that are managed well by her family with the help of the Palliative Care Home Team. The minister has come out to visit Dottie several times and she is grateful for her visits. She hasn't been able to get out to church yet, but she hasn't been hospitalized either. She is still hopeful that she will feel well enough to make it to church one of these Sundays. "Maybe when the weather is a little better." In the meantime, she loves her wheelchair and her home health aide, Luz, and she enjoys staying in her home of forty-five years.

## REFLECTIONS ON DOTTIE AND FAMILY

At this time, palliative care is a service that is very difficult for people to understand. Part of the reason is because it is not yet a consistently defined program like hospice care is. Most palliative care services are provided when people are hospitalized, like with Dottie.[1] Sometimes palliative care is provided as a home care program or in a nursing home, but it is not widely available outside the hospital. Palliative care consults are provided by doctors and other clinicians to people who have a serious illness and are often still opting for acute medical care, like hospitalization. Palliative care teams help families make decisions about future medical care they would want, such as resuscitation, and they specialize in managing distressing symptoms.[2] They focus on what's most important to people and how to match medical care with people's choices. It is not the same as hospice care, yet many people are confused about that, like Susan was.

Hospice care is for people who are in the final six months of life. They elect comfort measures only. This means that they choose to forgo tests, treatments, and hospitalization for their illness, and they allow the disease to advance as it normally would until death, with the support and expertise of the hospice care team.[3]

Both palliative care and hospice care are holistic in nature. This means that they focus on the whole person and their family, not just the illness. They help with physical symptoms, emotional reactions and coping, financial concerns, spiritual well-being, and the practical, day-to-day care that's needed when a family member has a serious or terminal illness.[4] Both programs work with other community services to provide additional help for people, such as transportation, food, and household chores. This was a big help, not only to Dottie but also to Janey and Susan.

Dottie made it really clear that she did not want to go back to the hospital unless she really needed to. No one really does. And yet, so many people who are elderly go back and forth to the hospital several times in a year. Like Dottie, they "don't want to live like that anymore!" There is a lot that people can do to understand symptoms, determine what some of the triggers are, and learn how to manage occurrences. Clear, written instructions on exactly what to do,[5] along with close guidance from medical providers, can be extremely helpful in preventing a crisis from unfolding.[6]

CHAPTER 3

# Good Days and Bad Days

My mother has lived a long, full, and accomplished life. She raised a large family, worked as a nurse for twenty years caring for people with disabilities, and somehow managed to sew, cook, travel, and play golf. If you have a question about how to launder a particular fabric, or what technique to use when rolling out piecrust, Mum is the one to ask. She has high standards and is fastidiously neat and organized. My mother is a traditionalist who was raised a devout Catholic but over time has come to realize that divorce, same-sex marriage, and couples living together before marriage are realities, and what is more important is that the people she loves are happy and healthy.

Mum is fiercely independent. Like many strong women of her generation, she does not like to rely on anyone to do her chores; besides, no one does as good a job as she does. My dad died twenty years ago, and Mum got used to doing things for herself. She loves her privacy, despite frequent visits and calls from her children, grandchildren, and now great-grandchildren. Mum spends her days reading, cleaning, putting together jigsaw puzzles, and watching TV, usually golf or the news.

One day, my mother asks all of her children to come over for a meeting. She is neatly dressed in her pink turtleneck and soft paisley pants with jewelry and shoes to match. She sits in her favorite accent chair in her large living room while my brothers and sisters settle into various seats around the room and on the floor. After a few minutes of the usual joking and bantering among my siblings, my mother presides over the family gathering like the matriarch she is.

Mum looks down at her hands, rubs the back of them, and then folds them in her lap and begins, "I've asked you all to come over so I can tell you about a decision I've made. I have decided to sign a DNR (Do Not Resuscitate) form." She looks around the room at everyone and continues, "I've lived a full life and I don't want to prolong it unnecessarily. Besides, the chances of my surviving resuscitation at my age and with my medical condition are almost nil."

My sister Nora is a palliative care doctor and Mum's health care proxy. We both had advance knowledge of this decision. My brother Peter wasn't so sure. "What if you are able to be resuscitated and get better?" he mildly contests. "Wouldn't that be worth it?"

Nora jumps in. "Mum is now ninety. She's had a heart attack and now has a pacemaker. She has high blood pressure, heart disease, and arthritis. Even if she was able to be resuscitated, she wouldn't be well enough to enjoy a good quality of life."

Mum agrees. "I don't want to go through what your father went through in the end. I don't want any of you to have to go through that either."

As I look around the room, it occurs to me that there are many different experiences and opinions about how my father's final days went. For my part, I was cross-country skiing in the middle of nowhere with my sisters Nora and Rose. We got a call at the cabin that my dad went into cardiac arrest and was unresponsive and on a respirator in the intensive care unit at the hospital. The plan was to discontinue, or "pull the plug" on, the respirator at 3 p.m. that day. I remember driving to the hospital, watching the clock in the car flash 3 p.m., wondering if my dad had died. He hadn't. When the respirator was disconnected, he breathed on his own for two more days before he died. Looking back, many of us felt that those two days gave everyone a chance to see him before he died. For one of my sisters, the sight of him having a seizure and the sound of the respirator will always stay with her. Many of us felt that he was finally at peace. Dad had had a stroke two years prior and endured many medical treatments, procedures, complications, and hospitalizations. He was not very happy. This had a big impact on my mother. She had a front-row seat to the change in my father's character and his will to live. Now, she wants some control over her own.

After a while, the family meeting resorts to the usual joking around. What is it they say about Irish families? "Funerals are happy occasions, and weddings are sad." We can joke about just about anything. In fact, many of us have health care experience, so we understand what Mum is saying to be true. Resuscitation at her age and in her condition would likely be traumatic and unsuccessful.[1] Soon, everyone says they are fine with it. After all, we know Mum is always clear about what she wants and doesn't want. There is never any doubt about that!

A few months after that meeting, we all start to get concerned. Whenever we visit, we notice bruises and occasionally skin tears on her arms and legs. A while back, Mum had been evaluated for dizziness and balance problems, but the doctor never found anything conclusive. Mum would always just wave off our concerns, saying, "Oh, I just bruise easily;

it's nothing." When the falls start to happen more frequently, our family decides to set up a schedule and take turns visiting Mum around suppertime to share a meal with her and help her get into bed for the night. She protests at first but then seems to enjoy the company and security.

Just two days shy of her ninety-second birthday, Mum is sitting on the side of her bed; she feels dizzy and her right arm and leg feel numb. Being a nurse, she knows something is wrong and calls 911. At the hospital, Mum is diagnosed with a mild stroke.

After her medical condition stabilizes, Nora and I research rehabilitation units for Mum to go to for intensive physical and occupational therapy. She regains full use of her right arm, but her right leg is still weak and she needs a walker to get around. The rehabilitation facility is a nice, old Victorian home. Mum has a large, sunny room to herself and her own bathroom. All the staff are cheerful, encouraging, and kind. Mum hates it. She thinks it is noisy, boring, and pointless. "So what, they watch me brush my teeth and walk up and down the hall with the walker; I don't need to be here to do that!"

Over time, it is clear that Mum's mental health is plummeting faster than her physical abilities are improving. At a care plan meeting at the rehabilitation facility with the staff, Mum, and a couple of my siblings, it is decided that Mum needs to leave. My youngest brother, Michael, and his family offer to have Mum move in with them for a while. They fix up a nice bedroom, bathroom, and sitting room for her. The rehabilitation staff make arrangements for her to have a hospital bed, wheelchair, and walker before she is discharged to Michael's home.

After this ordeal, Mum makes another decision: She does not want to go back to the hospital unless it is needed for comfort. Thankfully, we are all in complete agreement. We know what she just went through and are fully aware that she would not want that ever again. From this point on, Nora and I continue to talk with Mum about her wishes. At her request, we continue to insist on a comfort care plan, and we become Mum's fierce advocates for preventing unnecessary and burdensome health care procedures.

Over the next two years, Mum is cared for by a combination of family and hired nurse's aides. She becomes more infirm and is no longer able to walk. She needs help with all bathing, dressing, toileting, and mobility. She also develops macular degeneration of her eyes and is now hard of hearing. Mum can no longer read, sew, or do jigsaw puzzles. She has good days and bad days. On good days, she sits out on the porch and enjoys the sunshine and the birds that fly back and forth from the shrubs to the birdfeeder. She also loves seeing her great-grandchildren, especially the infants and toddlers. Mum has always had a knack for quieting a crying baby.

On bad days, Mum is angry and frustrated. She yells at caregivers, tells them they don't know what they are doing, and demands to know where all her belongings are. It is clear that she is dealing with a loss of control and grief, but any and all suggestions to help her either fail or are met with resistance. Mum is also sad and depressed. My oldest brother died of a heart attack when he was only fifty-three years old; this left Mum heartsick. Many of her friends and family members have also died. "I feel like I'm waiting for a catastrophic event," she says. Even though Mum's will to live is declining, her core strength and stamina are strong.

One beautiful, sunny Mother's Day, Mum and I are sitting out on the front porch watching the birds and squirrels swoop and scurry about. We begin to reminisce about the past. Being a mother also, I ask Mum what has been the hardest part about being a mother. "Losing Harold, of course, and also raising children during the 1960s. You never stop worrying about your children, no matter how old they are."

I agree. I tell Mum what so many patients I have cared for over the years have told me: "There's a terrible sense of wrong timing when a child dies before a parent. There's a deep sorrow that never goes away."

At the hospice where I am currently working, one of our patients has decided to voluntarily stop eating and drinking. I tell Mum a little bit about her story and then ask her, "Mum, would you ever consider doing that?"

Without hesitation, she says, "No. It's against my faith. I will go when the good Lord takes me."

As I sit there with my mother on Mother's Day, talking about being a mother, about life, death, and faith, my heart swells with gratitude for this time with her. I cherish this moment. This is one of our good days.

There continue to be good days and bad days. Every time I visit, I try to make Mum happy. I bring fresh soup, take her out to get her nails done, or buy her homemade jams and jellies. I offer to take her outside or read a book to her. Every time I drive back home, I feel empty. I can't really make her happy. Finally, a friend of mine tells me, "It's her process, not yours." It makes sense. Her grief and spiritual distress are not mine to solve. I can do little things to brighten her day, but it's mental health and spiritual counselors—and Mum herself—who can help with the biggest weights on Mum's soul. Yet the angst is shared.

After a period of several bad days with angry outbursts, sleepless nights, fired caregivers, and household stress, Michael calls a family meeting. He and his wife, Sally, can no longer manage Mum's care. "It's causing too much stress on my family and my job," he says. We totally understand and begin to look at nursing homes. We decide on a small nursing home in the next town over. It's another old, Victorian-type home that is clean and bright, and the staff seem friendly.

One afternoon, Michael and I have a talk with Mum. We even arrange to have an amplifier with headphones so she can easily hear everything we say. We are surprised when she indicates a willingness to go. Mum is adamant that she does not want her children to "give up their lives to care for her." She does not want to be a burden. After a brief visit and tour, Mum moves into Spruce Manor two weeks later.

For the most part, things go well at Spruce Manor. The large two-story home has big airy rooms and a beautiful front porch adorned with hanging plants. The staff are very engaging and compassionate. They clearly have expertise in caring for seniors, particularly people with dementia. The only consistently frustrating occurrence is that Mum's pillows and clothes seldom end up on her bed and in her drawers. Even though everything has her name on it, we end up gathering up her laundry from other people's rooms. For someone who is so particular about her laundry and pillows, it's maddening. However, when we talk with Mum about it, she doesn't want to make any waves. Is this the generational difference that I have lived with all my life, where my mother has deferred to authority and my sisters and I speak up? Or is Mum worried the nursing home staff will take it out on her if she complains? Probably a little bit of both.

Within the first month of living at Spruce Manor, Mum seems to decline mentally. Her affect is vague and she spends more time sleeping. She doesn't seem all that interested in anything anymore. Even though our family visits often, she is less social and appears more distant.

One Friday, on a beautiful, clear September day, I travel to Spruce Manor to visit Mum before going away for the weekend for my anniversary. When I arrive at the nursing home, I am shocked to see my mother from a distance. She is sitting in her wheelchair in the common area adjacent to the nurses' desk. She is dressed in her typical pastel turtleneck and matching elastic-waist pants, but she is slumped over; her hair is disheveled and her face looks pale and thin. My mother looks like a confused and frail nursing home patient!

"Hi, Mum, it's Reeny," I say as I kneel down in front of her. "How are you doing?"

Mum slowly lifts her head as I watch her sleepy eyes squint and try to focus.

"Are you doing okay, Mum? You seem awfully sleepy."

Mum doesn't answer. She lifts up her left arm and rests her elbow on the arm of the wheelchair, and her cheek on her fist. I glance over at the nurse, Karen, who says that Mum's been like this all morning. She assures me that she has not heard anything from the night nurses about whether Mum was up a lot during the night. She reports that Mum did not receive any sedatives last night or this morning.

"Mum, it's a beautiful day out. Would you like to go outside?"

There's no response. I shrug at Karen and then begin to gather Mum's sunglasses, water bottle, and sweater, and place them in her lap. I wheel her out to the patio on the left side of the home and carefully position her wheelchair up to the round cast-iron table. I brush off the seat of one of the chairs and sit down to Mum's left. I try to make conversation about this beautiful day and about various family updates. Again,

Mum barely responds to anything I say, so I ask her again, "Mum, what's going on? Why are you so sleepy?"

She looks up and in a matter-of-fact tone says, "Well, I'm going to die today."

Shocked by this, I think of all those heart-to-heart conversations I have had with hospice patients. Often they will say something profound, which is followed by a thoughtful pause, as I construct a response that seems accepting and neutral but mostly just encourages someone to talk more. "Are you okay with that, Mum?"

When she doesn't respond, I ask her, "Mum, have you had the Anointing of the Sick?"

No response. After a few seconds, she says, sounding mildly annoyed, "I don't know, Reeny. Check my record."

I smile because it seems like such a nurse thing to say. I look over at Mum. Her left hand rests on the table and her right hand is holding up her head again. I look closely at Mum's familiar hand. The skin looks loose over her boney knuckles and enlarged veins. She has pale pink nail polish on. I take a picture of her hand. My eyes well up thinking of all the holding, wiping, creating, and fixing these hands have done. I know that soon I will no longer be able to see these hands in real life anymore.

After a while I gather up her belongings and we go back inside. After settling her in, I kiss her goodbye. "I love you, Mum. See you soon." I tell Karen what Mum has said about dying today. Even though I doubt that she is going to die today, I tend to believe when people tell me things like that. I remind Karen that I will be away and that they should call Nora if there is a change in Mum's condition.

After I drive home, I call Nora and tell her about my visit. "Does she seem like she is in her final day to you?"

"No," I say. "She hasn't had a change in eating, nor does her color look that gray. She's definitely lethargic; I'm not sure why. Do you think we should call other family members and let them know?"

"Probably not. I'll check in with the staff later today and over the weekend," Nora says. "If anything changes, I'll be sure to let everyone know."

Mum didn't die that day. After a quiet weekend, she seems more alert. Several family members visit and they all report that she seems fine. Over the weekend, I try not to worry too much about Mum. This is another one of those times when it's nice to have a big family.

Two weeks later, in early October, Mum attends the wedding of my niece Jessica. When she arrives at the church, I notice that she has a slight cough and her nose is drippy. She keeps a tissue balled up on her lap and frequently wipes her nose and mouth. It's a chilly day near the ocean, but Mum is glad to be with everyone. She is all bundled up under a blanket and doted on by her children. By the time she arrives back at Spruce Manor, she is chilled and tired.

Two days later, Mum develops a fever, chills, and a terrible cough. She just can't warm up. Over the next two weeks, she has very little to eat or drink and she sleeps most of the time. Lots of family come to visit and take turns sitting at her bedside. One day, she is more awake and asks for a coffee milkshake, and another day, she is semiconscious and not talking at all. Some days it looks like she is going to get over this "bug," and other days, it seems clear she won't.

Soon it becomes obvious that Mum is dying. Our family sits at her bedside and cries, prays, laughs, and reminisces. The priest from the local church comes and anoints and blesses her. We all know that Mum is a very strong woman, so no one is surprised or impatient when Mum lives several weeks with very little to eat or drink. She doesn't appear to be waiting for anyone or anything. She has always had tremendous strength and stamina.

When Mum is in her final days of life, the staff at Spruce Manor move her into a private room. We take turns staying with her overnight. One night, Nora, Rose, and I are sitting at Mum's bedside talking and reminiscing. The staff come in often to offer us snacks and emotional support. We begin to notice that Mum's breathing is becoming more labored; she almost looks like she is hyperventilating. She is getting regular doses of morphine and lorazepam to keep her comfortable. Nora calls in the nurse, Karen, who gives Mum an extra dose of morphine to calm her breathing. She also brings in a fan to help circulate air.[2] Nora and I both know that sometimes people at the end of life have irregular breathing patterns. Sometimes breathing gets really fast, and other times it stops for short periods. Oxygen doesn't always help. It's hard to watch Mum breathe so fast. We keep asking Karen to keep up on the doses of morphine until finally her breathing looks more comfortable and relaxed. Soon Mum is resting peacefully. We all glance at each other with a sigh of relief.

Nora, Rose, and I are all camped out in chairs. We rearrange our pillows and blankets, trying to get comfortable. A candle is flickering on the mantelpiece overhead next to pictures of our dad and brother.

I start to wonder if Mum is having a hard time letting go. I know it can be hard sometimes for parents to leave their children. When it looks like Mum is getting close to dying, I begin to talk softly to her. "Mum, Dad and Harold are waiting for you. We'll be okay. Thank you for being such an amazing mum. We will see you in every sunset, every rainbow, and whenever we look out over the ocean." Within seconds, Mum's breathing starts to slow down and then it gently stops. Nora, Rose, and I all look at each other and then back at Mum. We then put our heads down on the bed and rest there for a few moments in silence.

After calling the family and packing up a few items from Mum's room, Nora, Rose, and I head back to the family home. By now, it is almost 8 a.m. Just as we are getting out of our cars, we look up over the homestead and are touched by the sight of a beautiful rainbow encircling the sky. Mum is home.

### REFLECTIONS ON MUM AND FAMILY

Talking about DNR and other medical decisions is a sensitive topic among family members. Many people don't want to "talk like that," thinking that it will "upset people." They also don't want to acknowledge that death will eventually come. Some people worry that talking about end-of-life goals and treatment plans will take away someone's sense of hope, but that has not been found to be true.[3] In reality, these conversations are a relief to many people and are extremely helpful for family members and medical professionals to have.[4] These conversations clarify what various procedures mean and what someone would want for future medical care, and they help avoid important decision-making during stressful and emergency situations.[5] It was important for Mum to select a health care proxy who would carry out her wishes if she couldn't communicate them herself.[6] Most people are not fully awake in the final days of life. Having a health care proxy who would make decisions consistent with Mum's wishes was a relief to her.

Mum was very independent and didn't want to be a burden on others. Like many people her age, she had various aches and pains, and ups and downs. Over time, she had changes in her eyesight, hearing, mobility, and memory. The loss of these abilities, along with profound grief, dramatically impacted her quality of life. The "will to live" can be very strong but also seems to be lost when people don't feel that their life is fulfilling or meaningful anymore.

I agree with Dr. Ira Byock, hospice physician and consultant, who says,

> At both poles of life, as we are born and as we die, we will be physically dependent on others. We don't consider the absolute physical dependence and vulnerability and even incontinence of infants and toddlers as being anything abnormal or undignified, and yet, at the end of life we're supposedly undignified because we're physically dependent on others and even incontinent. I think at both poles of life, caring for one another is what we do. That is, in fact, part of our very humanity. Being ill and physically dependent on others at the end of life doesn't make one undignified, it simply makes one human.[7]

Mum, and everyone else, deserves that.

## CHAPTER 4

# When Is Active Treatment No Longer Worth It?

Lena sits back and admires her yard. June has always been her favorite time of year—warm but not too hot. Large maple and oak trees shade the yard and various shrubs line the back edge of the property. Lilies, dahlias, and hydrangeas bloom in soothing shades of pink and blue. Thick, manicured grass wraps around the flower beds, giving the yard a lush, park-like feeling. A statue of the blessed mother is nestled in among the flowers. Lena bows her head, closes her eyes, and says a short prayer. She checks her watch and then walks quickly toward the back stairs of the house.

"Stan!" she calls, gently closing the screen door behind her. Stanislaw usually takes his morning nap until noontime. Lena has prepared his lunch already. She wants to be sure he is done and changed before a nurse comes over at 1 p.m. today.

Lena walks through the kitchen and into the spacious living room. There, Stan is in his recliner, just waking up. "Well, hello, honey, time for some lunch." Stan arches his back, straightens out his arms, and yawns. His polo shirt and gray sweatpants are twisted over his small frame. Lena reaches down and puts his sneakers on and tightens the Velcro straps. She moves his wheelchair right up against the recliner and says, "Ready?" As she has done so many times before, she helps Stan stand, quickly changes his diaper, helps him pivot, and then guides him safely into his wheelchair. She unlocks the chair and carefully wheels him up to the kitchen table.

Lena opens the refrigerator and grabs the egg salad sandwich and cup of milk and puts it on the table. She tucks a hand towel into the front of his shirt collar and drapes it over his lap.

"Here you go!" she says as she slides the sandwich and cup up to her husband. Lena reaches over and grabs her morning coffee cup. There's still half a cup left, so she puts it in the microwave and then reaches into the refrigerator and grabs the bowl with the rest of the egg salad. She takes a deep breath, rubs her lower back, and sits at the table across from Stan.

All of a sudden, Lena feels a pang of fear rise up in her chest as she remembers the nurse will be here shortly. She thinks back to Stan's recent doctor's appointment. The blood test showed that he is anemic; plus he has lost fifteen pounds in the past year. She knows he's lost weight. She can tell just by helping him wash and move around. His clothes hang off of him. Stan was diagnosed with Alzheimer's disease a year and a half ago. Since then, he has lost more independence and depends more on Lena for his day-to-day care. The doctor said he would like a nurse from the Visiting Nurses and Hospice Agency to come over and evaluate him. "Stan, keep eating your sandwich, sweetheart. Take another bite," Lena says as she sips her coffee and reaches for her notepad and pencil. Stan looks up blankly through his black-framed glasses and returns to his meal. Lena reviews her grocery list and then jots down: pads, wipes, milk.

She glances up at the clock and then jumps up, gently wipes Stan's mouth and hands with a napkin, and then carefully folds up the corners of the towel that was tucked under his chin, in order to keep crumbs and egg pieces inside. Stan looks down at the table expressionless as Lena places a fidget spinner in his hand. She gulps her last sip of coffee as she quickly loads the dishes in the dishwasher.

She's only had enough time to brush her hair and put on some lipstick when the doorbell rings. Lena opens the door and greets two women. The shorter woman with long, curly hair introduces herself as Charlene, the hospice nurse, and her taller, athletic-looking colleague is Pat, a social worker. Lena welcomes them both in and offers them tea and some cookies. "What a beautiful home you have," Charlene says as she follows Lena through the living room toward the kitchen.

"Oh, thank you. Stanislaw and I live on the first floor, and our tenant lives upstairs."

Pat immediately notices that everything about their home is meticulous. The living room is spacious, clean, and organized. The walls are full of photographs, knickknacks, religious relics, and mementos. Furniture is neatly arranged around the living room.

Charlene and Pat both greet Stanislaw and introduce themselves. He looks up but doesn't respond. After some small talk, they settle in and start the evaluation.

"Tell us a little bit about Stanislaw and yourself," Charlene begins. "Where were you raised?"

"We were both born in the Old Country. We moved from Poland just after we were married, in 1952. His older brother was already living here, so we moved in with him at first."

"What sort of activities have you both enjoyed?" Pat asks, glancing at Stanislaw and then Lena.

"We are both members of the Polish American Club and Sacred Heart Church. Stan used to be in the choir. We both used to love going to the Annual Polish Festival, right, honey?"

Lena smiles as she remembers him dancing to polka music, his legs skipping side to side, his arms pumping up and down. "We both loved the home-cooked food, friends, music, and dancing. We haven't been able to go for the last couple of years, but our friends from the church have brought us some galumpkis and pierogies from the fair. It's been hard getting Stan out of the house now. Usually I have to call for the senior center van; it's a big ordeal."

"Well, let's talk about Stan's situation and what's involved in his care," Charlene begins. Over the next half an hour, Lena gives Charlene and Pat a detailed picture of all the care she provides to Stan and how things have changed over time. What becomes clear to both of them is that the care that Lena gives Stan is as organized and meticulous as their house and yard. Lena shares her detailed strategy and system for every aspect of his care, from padding the bed, to helping him shower, to preparing his meals. She wakes him up in the morning, transfers him to a wheelchair, gives him his medications, feeds him breakfast, helps him shower or sponge bathe, and then, while he naps, tends to the house, yard, bills, and all else. When Charlene suggests that Lena also "take care of herself too," Lena waves her hand away, smiles very slightly, and then changes the subject back to Stan.

"A couple of times I have had to call our tenant Walter upstairs for help getting him into the van. Unfortunately, both of our children live out of state, so I have had to rely on help from neighbors and friends from the church. Walter sits with Stan once or twice a week so I can do my shopping and errands. He mostly just sleeps when I'm gone. In fact, he sleeps most of the time anyway. He hasn't really said more than a couple of words in the past several months." Lena looks over at Stan, who is looking down and tugging on his sweatpants.

Charlene reaches over and puts the fidget spinner from his lap back into his hands.

"Lena, can you tell me a little bit about Stanislaw's medical history?"

Lena reaches over and grabs a notebook from the shelf underneath the kitchen counter. The notebook is adorned with red, pink, and white flowers. Lena uses the string at the bottom of the notebook to open it. She flips back a few sheets from the bookmarked page and begins to give a report of Stan's hospitalizations and dates, his current medication list, and the medical supplies he currently uses. Once again, Charlene and Pat look at each other, smile, and tell Lena, "You're amazing."

"Well, I'm just trying to keep track of everything." Lena looks down at her lap, takes a deep breath, twirls her rings, and says, "The last time we went to the doctor's, he said that Stan has anemia. They said he'll have to get blood tests all the time, and if his blood count is low, he'll need a transfusion. I can't even imagine getting him out that many times. I'm worried; without a ramp or an extra person, it will be difficult to get him to the hospital."

"It sounds very difficult," Pat agrees. "That's one of the reasons why your doctor asked us to come out and do an evaluation and talk with you. It helps us to understand what stage his Alzheimer's disease is at and what level of care he needs."

"What about when it's winter? What would I do then?" Lena says as she reaches for a tissue and blots the corners of her eyes. Charlene reaches over and gently rubs Lena's upper arm. Lena looks over at Stan, who is starting to doze off. With Charlene's help, they transfer Stan back into his recliner and then return to the kitchen with Pat.

Once they're seated back at the table, Pat continues, "Lena, at this point in his life, what do you think is most important, or most enjoyable, to Stan?"

"Well, even though he's confused and doesn't recognize people anymore, I think he knows he's home. He doesn't really talk at all, but sometimes he mumbles some words in Polish, especially when he's dozing. He's in a routine of eating, bathing, and sleeping. We've been managing okay. He seems to like it when I put polka music on or when we watch mass on the television."

"You've been managing remarkably well," Pat says. "You take wonderful care of Stan. Charlene and I are both amazed at your system and recordkeeping."

They all weave a conversation around stories of the past, various recent incidents, and what this new anemia diagnosis means in the long run. Charlene and Pat explain that his dementia will continue to get worse. There actually is a predictable pattern of decline that happens to people with dementia.[1] There are even charts that explain the typical decrease in eating, toileting, moving around, and talking that happens over time.[2] Unfortunately, there are also many complications that often happen to people with dementia, such as aspiration pneumonia, falls, and skin problems. "It can be scary to look ahead, but most people find it helpful to understand what's happening," Charlene explains.

With tears welling up in her eyes, Lena says, "Stan wouldn't want to keep getting blood transfusions. He's happy being home." Lena wipes her eyes, blows her nose, and straightens out her skirt. "I don't want to do anything to hurt him, though," Lena adds quickly.

"Of course you don't, Lena," Pat reassures her. "This is a difficult situation. It's hard to know what to do. Lena, we will be reporting back to the doctor that Stan's dementia is pretty advanced. This means that because he has lost so much weight, isn't able to walk or use the toilet, and doesn't really speak, he is likely already eligible for hospice care because of his dementia. The doctor is the one who actually decides this based on his medical condition and our report. But if he agrees, it means that his prognosis is probably only six months or so. I know this is hard to hear, but this might impact how you think about and plan for this new information about his anemia."

Lena sighs deeply. "Well, this is a lot to take in. Let me talk with my boys."

"Of course. We're going to leave you with these brochures. If either of your children want to talk with us directly, please feel free to pass along our phone numbers. We'll send a report to Stan's doctor and then they'll follow up with you."

After seeing Charlene and Pat out, Lena pauses to look at Stan, who's sleeping peacefully in his recliner. His head is back and his mouth is open. His cheekbones look even more pronounced.

"Dear God, please be with us," Lena says as she wipes her eyes. Lena returns to the kitchen, grabs some potatoes, and begins to peel them at the sink.

Back in the car, Charlene turns to Pat. "What a wonderful couple," she says. "It's so heart-wrenching. It's amazing how many decision points there are at various medical intersections when people have a serious or terminal illness. People need so much information and clarification, on so many levels, in order to make decisions that they're comfortable with."

Charlene passes along her report to the hospice medical director and hematologist. After a follow-up conference with

Stan's family and doctors, he is referred for hospice care. Everyone is in agreement that forgoing treatment for Stan's anemia is the best decision for everyone. Lena is relieved.

Over the next three months, hospice visits regularly with Stan and Lena. At weekly nursing visits, Lena carefully reviews his eating and toileting history. She crosses off a list of questions asked and medical supplies ordered. Charlene gives suggestions about skin care, bowel-regulation medications, and eating tips. "People in Stan's condition are at risk for aspiration pneumonia," Charlene explains. "Because his swallowing ability is decreasing, it's important to make sure that food doesn't go down the wrong pipe. Food going into the lungs, instead of the stomach, is what often causes aspiration pneumonia."[3] Charlene explains the many ways that Lena can reduce Stan's risk of aspirating.[4]

"What about those supplement drinks or shakes—would those help him?"

"They might," Charlene says. "You can always try them and see if he likes it. Just make sure you only give him a small amount at a time." Lena carefully writes down all the instructions.

During another routine check-in visit, Lena tells Charlene that Stan has developed a rash on both sides of his groin. She walks quickly into the bathroom and returns showing Charlene a tube of ointment. "I've tried putting this diaper rash cream on it, but it hasn't helped any."

Lena and Charlene walk together into Stan's bedroom where he is sleeping on his back in the hospital bed. Charlene notices that Stan's cheeks and collarbones seem more prominent, likely due to his continued weight loss. Stan is dressed in a gray T-shirt with the words "Best Dziadzio" written in red letters with the Polish flag beneath them. "It means 'grandfather' in Polish," Lena explains. "It was a gift from his grandson, John." When Lena turns down the sheet covering Stan, he has on just a diaper and gray athletic socks. Again, Charlene notices that his legs look pale and thin, and his kneecaps look large and knobby. Lena gently peels apart the adhesive tabs on his diaper and points out the rash to Charlene.

Charlene washes her hands, puts on gloves, and carefully examines the pink skin areas on his groin and the inner part of his upper legs. "It looks like it could be a fungus rash; it's very common, especially in moist areas like the groin." Charlene also does her usual assessment, looking at the rest of his skin and listening to his lungs and belly. Stan sleeps peacefully through the visit. After conferring with the doctor, Charlene makes arrangements for an antifungal cream to be delivered to their home the next day. Lena reaches for her pad of paper and writes it all down.

One day, Lena is in the living room getting ready to transfer Stan into the wheelchair for lunch. "Honey, are you ready?" she says once the wheelchair is lined up diagonally with the recliner. Stan's eyes are open, but his expression is blank. Lena helps him to stand, but just as she is about to have him turn and sit in the wheelchair, Stan's knees buckle and he slides down onto the floor. He is sitting up but his back is leaning sideways against the recliner and his legs are bunched up in front of him. "Oh my God, sweetheart! Are you okay? Are you hurt?"

Lena can feel her heart racing. She tries to push up Stan's torso so he is sitting more upright, but he just leans back again. "Help! Walt! Are you up there?" Lena yells.

Within seconds, she hears footsteps barreling down the stairs. Walter, her tenant, bursts into the living room and runs over to Lena and Stan. He straightens Stan's legs, manages to get behind him, and bear-hugs him up and into the chair. "Are you okay, my friend?" Walter asks him as he kneels down in front of Stan. No response. "That was pretty scary, but you seem okay now," Walter reassures them.

"I'm so sorry I had to call you down. Thank God you were home. I don't know what I would have done!"

Lena anxiously tidies up the side table and profusely apologizes for the "imposition," while Walter reassures them, "It was no trouble, really."

Lena wheels Stan up to the kitchen table for lunch. With her hands still shaking, she reaches over and grabs Charlene's card and calls the hospice number. The receptionist tells her that the hospice team is just finishing their weekly meeting. Once Charlene comes on the phone, Lena begins to recount the incident. "Stan slipped down from the recliner onto the floor while I was trying to transfer him into the wheelchair. My neighbor helped get him back into the chair," she says with her voice loud and quick, then adds, "How do I know if he's hurt?" Charlene reassures her that she will come right over and check him out.

When Charlene arrives, Stan is sitting in his wheelchair in his bedroom with light blue pajamas on. His shoulders are slouched and his head is bent forward slightly. His chin has a slight stubble of a beard that he rubs with the back of his hand. "Hello, Stan, it's Charlene, your nurse." His eyes are open, but they don't follow Charlene's voice. "I'm going to check to make sure you're okay and nothing is hurting you."

Charlene then begins to assess Stan. He is able to move his legs and feet without showing signs of pain, and he doesn't seem to have any cuts or bruises anywhere. She checks his vital signs and then reassures Lena, "I think he's okay for now." Charlene then explains to Lena what to look for in terms of nonverbal signs of pain or discomfort and ways to prevent falls. As usual, she also compliments Lena on her impeccable care. She knows that sometimes when these complications happen, Lena expresses regret and worry that she isn't doing enough or that she did something wrong. "You're amazing, Lena," Charlene tells her. "It's a difficult job, but you're doing wonderfully caring for him."

"Thank you so much, Charlene, for coming over so quickly. My sons are so grateful that I have hospice to call night or day whenever something like this happens."

"Absolutely, Lena. That's what we're here for; you're not alone in this. We do have additional help we can offer you, Lena. We can have a home health aide come out and help you with bathing Stan. We could also arrange a respite stay for Stan if you feel that you need a break from his care for a few days."

"No, I don't think so, Charlene. I'm all set for now. It was just very scary to see him on the floor like that. I think I'll just stick with my visits from you and Pat for now. The priest from Sacred Heart is coming over tomorrow, so that will help."

Stan and Lena have a routine, and they're managing. There are always ups and downs. Charlene and Pat continue to visit them and teach Lena what to expect as Stan's condition worsens and he gets closer to dying. They also continue to support her and praise the care she provides to Stanislaw. Lena knows she can always call whenever anything comes up. In the meantime, Stan and Lena enjoy the time they have left together. Every day after breakfast, she puts on polka music, and the mood in their spacious apartment seems to lift a little. Every evening after supper, she puts on the television and relaxes for a bit while Stan dozes off to sleep.

## REFLECTIONS ON STANISLAW AND FAMILY

Many diseases, like Alzheimer's disease, have predictable patterns as someone's condition gets worse. There are telltale signs that someone is in the final stage of life.[5] Hospice and palliative care clinicians are not only very aware of these signs but are also required by Medicare and other insurance companies to compare a person's condition to these "end-stage signs" in order to show that someone is eligible for hospice.[6] It can be hard for loved ones, like Lena, to see changes over time and to know these signs. Palliative and hospice care clinicians can help explain these stages to families, which often helps them make difficult medical decisions.

There are so many people who are in the same situation as Stanislaw and Lena. Providing care to a loved one can be emotional and isolating. Family members are often accustomed to providing bedside personal care, but the medical side of care is often unknown and stressful. As in Lena's case, it can be difficult to make decisions about whether to treat a disease when someone is in the final stages of life. It can be an added weight when the decision is being made by a family member for someone else. The decision to keep with a "treatment-focused plan of care" versus a "comfort-care-only plan of care" often comes down to how much longer someone is expected to live and whether the person and/or loved one wants to pursue hospitalization going forward.[7] The decision often involves looking at what medical testing and treatments are recommended, balanced with questions about how taxing it would be for someone to endure. Would it be worth it? Would it cause more harm than good? These questions are often best answered by focusing on the person and determining who they are and what they would want.

CHAPTER 5

# How Long Does Mom Have to Live?

Her name at birth and christening was Wilma Mae Robinson, but everyone calls her "Mama." Her daughter Shanice remembers their small, green ranch home was the center of the neighborhood universe. Everyone played at Mama's house, with her six children, two dogs, and an endless number of adventures waiting. Summer days were spent playing baseball, fishing, jumping off the roof of the shed, or cooling off in the sprinkler. Mama always sat out on her porch, reading the newspaper or church bulletin, or peeling something for dinner. Her loose dress formed a cloth basket in her lap that she used for holding food, sewing, or comforting young children.

Mama is a woman of faith. Every Sunday was spent getting dressed up and attending worship service at the Black Baptist church. After the service, everyone would gather at Mama's house for fellowship and a feast. Shanice can picture her mama cooking in the kitchen, wearing a full bib apron, and humming the hymns from the morning's service. Mama models the acceptance and compassion of the Baby Jesus. Every word of gratitude ends with "praise the Lord with all my heart." Shanice, her brothers and sisters, and the neighbors' children all feel this divine gift in the form of being loved.

Now Wilma is eighty-two years old and just back from the hospital after having a stroke that left her paralyzed on her right side and unable to talk. A hospital bed has been moved into her small bedroom. She lies on her back with several layers of sheets and blankets underneath her from the ambulance. She seems to sense her family around her; everyone is getting updated, making calls, finding supplies, and helping her settle in. Wilma closes her eyes and settles into the familiar sounds and smells of home.

The living room is full of family members, talking to and ribbing each other, as siblings often do. Jamal, Wilma's oldest son, is catching good-natured heat for his Raiders cap. The rest of his brothers have long been New York Giants fans. Shanice smiles indulgently at her brothers while keeping an eye out for the hospice team to arrive.

A small red Jeep pulls up to the curb. Shanice meets two women at the door who introduce themselves as Charlene, the hospice nurse, and Carole, the spiritual counselor. Shanice leads them down the hallway and into the back bedroom. Earlier, her brothers rearranged the small space as best they could, shifting the dresser, two chairs, and a commode to one side of the room to accommodate the hospital bed. Shanice introduces Charlene and Carole to her sister, Gloria, and her niece, Maya, who are standing at the bedside.

"Mama." Shanice strokes her cheek. Her mama stares at the ceiling and shows no sign of recognition. Her face is smooth, as if all the creases of worry and joy have been erased by the stroke. Her head is wrapped in her familiar scarf, the black-and-purple one with geometric patterns. "This is Charlene and Carole from hospice. They're going to help us care for you."

The television on the wall, opposite the hospital bed, is tuned to the local news. Shanice is briefly distracted by the weatherman, who is pointing at a colorful map as if it's an ordinary day—chance of a late-afternoon thunderstorm, he says.

Charlene approaches Mrs. Robinson's left side, introduces herself, and asks her directly if she is having any pain or discomfort. She blinks but otherwise doesn't respond or move. Charlene asks the circle of women at the bedside if they think she is uncomfortable. In unison, they all shake their head or say no.

Maya, who is a nurse, explains what's been going on. "After Mama had her stroke, we didn't think she was going to make it." Maya pauses. "But slowly she seemed to become more awake. After a week in the hospital, she was transferred to a rehabilitation unit for physical therapy and speech therapy. That didn't go so well."

Shanice reaches for Mama's hand. "She hasn't been able to move her right arm or leg at all. Then she developed a urinary tract infection and ended up back in the hospital."

"She was very confused and restless at first," Maya adds. "When she got better, we all knew that we just wanted her to come home."

"Well," Carole says, "I think she knows she is home and surrounded by a lot of love. I'll leave you to tend to her while I go out and talk with the rest of your family."

The four women, two on each side, carefully turn Mama onto her side to remove the bulky sheets and blankets from beneath her. Charlene notices that Mama's right arm and leg are swollen; her dark brown skin is shiny and stretched taut, and a patch of skin on her tailbone is red. "It's important to turn her off her back every couple of hours and apply some barrier cream to any red spots." Maya reaches into one of the white plastic bags from the hospital and passes a tube of cream to Charlene. "We want to make sure her skin stays closed," she says.

As they all work together to wash Mama, apply barrier cream, loosely fasten a diaper, turn her, and smooth out her bed, they talk with her to explain what they're doing and give her gentle reassurance. "We're almost done, Mama." They turn her onto her good side and cushion her so that her paralyzed arm and leg are resting softly on pillows. "We'll let you rest now, Mama."

Gloria stays with Mama while Shanice, Maya, and Charlene move into the kitchen to continue talking. The kitchen walkway is narrow and lined with gold appliances and light brown cabinets. Leftovers from the family lunch—pizza boxes, paper plates, napkins, and drinks are stacked on the stove and countertop. Shanice clears a pile of papers from the small, round table, and the three of them sit down. Maya points to the pictures covering the wall—family weddings, school pictures of grandchildren, and a large portrait of the entire family taken two years ago when Mama turned eighty. "That was such a great day," Maya says.

Carole comes in from the living room and joins them at the table. "Is that your mama's Bible there?" Carole asks as she points to a black Bible with a single gold cross on the cover.

"Oh yes, Mama's prized Bible." Shanice smiles. "Every morning, without fail, Mama would read from her 'good book.' "

"It looks well-read," Carole says. "I'd be happy to visit for prayer or to read passages to her, if you'd like."

"Well, thank you, Carole. Folks from the church have been coming over every Sunday, even before all this happened. Her minister went to see her at the hospital, and Jamal has already called to let him know she's home. We have a lot of family, neighbors, and the church," Shanice says. "We're blessed."

They go on to talk about Mama: who she is, how she raised them, and what matters to her—family and faith. Charlene takes out a notebook and pen from her bag and starts to take notes. Shanice begins, "Mama has only been able to take a little bit of baby food, but that's it. They talked to us about a feeding tube at the hospital, but we decided not to get one."

Maya agrees. "I've taken care of people with feeding tubes, and I don't think Mama would want that. Besides, she seems to like the pureed peaches and bananas."

"You probably know this already," Charlene says, "but preventing aspiration is particularly important for your mama right now. Make sure she's awake and alert and raise the head of the bed up when you feed her. Also, liquids should be thickened as it makes it easier to swallow."[1] Charlene reaches into her bag and finds some packets of gelatin. She passes them to Shanice. "These will help with that."

As they all go back and forth talking about Mama, the important aspects of her care, and what to expect regarding hospice services, the sky darkens. "It looks like the storm is coming," Shanice says, pointing to the sliding glass door. Charlene rips out a page from her notebook where she has written down instructions for the family and begins to pack the notebook away in her bag.

"Before you go," Shanice asks nervously, "can I just ask you a question?" She darts a glance at her niece Maya. "Do you have a sense of how long she has to live?"

Charlene folds her hands on the table and calmly looks at Shanice and Maya. "Of course. Please ask us anything. This is probably the most common question we are asked."

Charlene shares the information about prognosis that she has shared many times before. "Hospice doesn't do anything to prolong or shorten a person's life," she explains. "Each day, we help to care for and support people until they die. As someone's disease gets worse, the person eats less, moves around less, and sleeps more. The final stages of life are marked by certain signs and symptoms. Hospice often uses terms such as 'actively dying' and 'imminently dying' to refer to the final weeks and days of someone's life."[2]

Shanice listens intently and wonders where Mama is at. Maya reaches over to hold Shanice's hand.

Charlene continues. "When someone begins their active dying phase, usually in the last week or two of life, they eat very little and mostly stay in bed. They sleep a lot, and even when they are awake, they seem distant or dreamlike.[3] Sometimes I refer to it as 'in between worlds.' Sometimes people 'time travel' and talk about when they were little. They may even talk to parents, siblings, and people from the past and say that they see people we can't see.[4] At this stage, they appear to be semiconscious and confused at times. The focus is to make sure the person is calm, comfortable, and safe."

In the final days and hours of life, people are generally not eating or drinking at all, and they are often unresponsive, meaning not awake. As before, the goal is to keep people comfortable and calm by managing any symptoms that might arise.[5]

"It seems to me that your mama could be entering her actively dying phase," Charlene gently tells them. "She's not eating very much, and she'll likely spend more of the day sleeping. Hospice will be with you through this process and will support your family, as you wish, every step of the way."

Shanice grabs a tissue. "That's kind of what we thought," she says. "It just helps us to have an idea."

Maya wraps her arms around her aunt as Shanice blots her eyes. "All of our lives will change forever," Shanice says through her tears, "but we must do what Mama would want us to do when she is back in the hands of her creator: Praise the Lord with all our heart!"

## REFLECTIONS ON WILMA AND FAMILY

Determining prognosis is not an exact science. Many people surpass all prognosis expectations. Other times, people die much sooner than expected. There are a lot of variables, both unique to an individual and in terms of diseases and complications.[6] When someone dies naturally, no one really knows exactly when that person will leave this world. However, hospice walks this walk with many people over time. They've come to see and understand what typically happens in these final stages of someone's life. Understanding these changes can help families, like Wilma's, prepare for each phase and know what care is needed at various stages.

Many African American families, like Wilma's, have strong ties to a community of faith. These are tremendous strengths that often form the basis of a family's "rules and themes" that they live by. Themes such as "it's in God's hands" or "that's what families are for" are often passed down from generation to generation and form guiding principles that help families during times of grief, sadness, and death.[7] Many families have their own caregivers, religious support, and built-in support system. This is particularly true for families of color. Often what is needed is a trusting relationship with health providers and expert medical guidance. Hospice is available to help with whatever is needed. It is also there to support what a family naturally does to care for a loved one who is sick and/or dying.

CHAPTER 6

# From Discord to Harmony

Ruth can usually be found sitting by the sunny window of the nursing home, stroking her stuffed dog, Barney. She has an infectious, toothless grin. Ruth has always loved the color red. Her closet is full of red blouses and sweaters. Her hands, now gnarly with arthritis, always have bright red nail polish painted on them by one of her granddaughters, who visit her regularly.

Ruth has lived at Maple Village Nursing Home for the past four years. She is well-known and loved by everyone. When she arrived, she was eighty-five years old and had moderate dementia. However, she was still able to walk around, participate in social activities, and engage with the staff and other residents. She was an avid bingo player and loved participating in the music and exercise programs. Ruth was able to recite prayers and songs in Hebrew and participate in Sabbath day activities.

Over the years, Ruth has become increasingly confused and frail. She started to have difficulty swallowing liquids, so the nurse practitioner requested a speech therapy consult and ordered thickened liquids. Ruth also had a fall when she slid from her bed onto the floor. She now has a cushion on the floor alongside her bed for protection. Her usual toothless grin has turned into a distressed facial expression with furrowed eyebrows, squinted eyes, and a clenched jaw. When she is bathed, she cries out, especially when the staff turn her over to change her diaper.

Ruth has two adult daughters who are very involved in her care. Rachel, the oldest, lives nearby and visits her mom two to three times a week after work. She works as a mortgage loan officer at a local bank. When she arrives at Maple Village, she greets the evening staff with a smile and warm but tired eyes. "How'd today go? How much of her breakfast and lunch did she eat?" Rachel always expresses thanks to the staff; she is grateful for their care and feels like they are working together on behalf of her mom. After talking with the nurse and aide, Rachel goes into her mom's room, takes off her suit jacket, pulls up a chair, and moves the overbed tray closer to her mom. She bends over, kisses her mom on her forehead, and says. "Hi, Mom, it's Rachel. I have a nice supper here for you."

Rachel is Ruth's health care proxy. She is adamant that Ruth be kept comfortable and not subjected to any unnecessary tests or hospitalizations. She doesn't want her mother to have any aggressive medical procedures or to be forced to participate in any activities that she doesn't seem to enjoy. She feels that hospitalization should be avoided at all costs. She knows her mom would be very disoriented in another setting and that it might even make things worse. Rachel has signed consents against hospitalization, resuscitation, and the use of any antibiotics. She feels that this cycle of infections and antibiotics will just prolong her mother's illness, and will do little to improve her quality of life.

Ruth's younger daughter, Leah, lives two hours away. She visits her mom at least every other weekend and sometimes more often if she can. Leah works at a school as a special education aide for a young boy who has multiple disabilities.

When Leah visits her mom, she comes into the hall at least every fifteen minutes and asks the staff for seemingly endless requests, "Can my mom have some juice with thickener? Can someone please come in and help get her up into the chair? When is she scheduled to have a shower?" The Maple Village nurses and aides try to attend to Leah's requests, but they are usually short-staffed on the weekends and Leah tries their patience. Leah moves around her mom's room, nervously straightening things up, throwing disposable cups and napkins away, and asking her mom, "Mom, what do you want to eat?"

Leah has always had a tense relationship with her sister, Rachel. She feels that Rachel treats her like an incompetent younger sister and never values her input. Both Leah and Rachel feel that they have a good relationship with their mom and have her best interest at heart. Their father died fifteen years ago of a stroke. The death was particularly difficult for Leah. As the "baby" of the family, she was close to her dad and his death left a big hole in her heart. She does not want to lose her mother. Rachel considers Leah to be emotional and impractical.

The nursing home staff has contacted Rachel several times in the past three months to report changes in Ruth's condition: infections, red skin areas, skin tears, and falls. Rachel thanks them for the call and then reiterates that she is forgoing hospitalization in favor of comfort-focused care. Rachel requests that they just keep her comfortable.

One Friday afternoon, the nursing home social worker, Jamie, coordinates a patient care conference with Rachel and Leah to discuss their mom's care. Rachel arrives hurriedly, in a bright blue business suit, and apologizes for being a few minutes late. Leah is already seated, talking calmly with Jamie about her job. Rachel goes over to Leah, gives her a loose hug, and takes the seat across from Jamie.

"Thank you both for coming; I know it's not easy on a weekday, but I appreciate your taking the time to meet. Please, help yourself to some cookies and a drink," Jamie begins. "The goal of this meeting is to discuss the changes that are happening with your mom and, hopefully, come together on a plan for her care. Is that okay with you both? Is that what you expected?"

Leah and Rachel both glance at each other. Rachel responds, "Yes."

Leah shrugs and nods, "I guess."

"Okay, as you know, your mom has been declining. She hasn't been eating as much as she used to, and she continues to lose weight. She's also having more periods of confusion and yelling out. I know the staff have talked with you both, at different times, about what's going on. I thought it might be helpful to have an open dialogue about her care, now and for the future. The staff has voiced concern that you two might be looking for different approaches to handling her medical needs and day-to-day activities."

Leah leans forward, tucks her curly hair behind her ears, and begins, "I only can come here about every other weekend. Every time I arrive, the lunch tray is on her table and the staff is nowhere to be found. Of course she's losing weight."

"Leah, the staff are feeding her," Rachel says. "I'm here three times a week. I'm sure the weekends are more difficult, but they are very attentive to Mom. You can't keep giving the staff a hard time. Mom is having a harder time with lots of things, not just eating. She can't hold her head up like she used to, and she's sleeping a lot more."

"I'm not 'giving the staff a hard time,' Rachel," Leah says. "I'm just asking them to do their job, that's all. I'm just looking out for Mom, who can't speak up for herself. She deserves the best care possible. Why can't they give her IV fluid?"

"We all know that you both want what's best for your mom," Jamie begins to explain. "Regular IV fluids do not replace the nutrition and fluids that people eat and drink."[1]

Rachel jumps in, "Leah, we're not doing that. Don't you remember the last time Mom was in the hospital? She had terrible bruising and pain from IVs. She also went into fluid overload on her heart from too much IV fluid.[2] She gets all confused and disoriented at the hospital. It's just not worth it!" Rachel sits back in her chair, closes her eyes, and takes a deep breath. "Look, all these seemingly minor treatments all come with a cost. Antibiotics have caused her rashes, stomachaches, and diarrhea. Everything just seems too risky for someone in Mom's condition. Leah, Mom is coming toward the end of her life and we both will need to come to terms with that."

"Mom is not dying!" Leah blurts out, her face red and her eyes narrowed. "I can't believe you're just going to do nothing and let her suffer!"

"No, Leah, quite the opposite. I'm trying to prevent her from suffering!"

Jamie tries to pull them together. "These are very difficult and emotional things to talk about. It's not uncommon for family members to have differing perspectives and opinions on how to handle things. Let's focus, for now, on some immediate situations and solutions for your mom's care." Jamie is successful in shifting the tension in the meeting toward addressing mealtime routines, helpful strategies, and the family's engagement with the staff. They all agree to talk again by phone in two weeks. They say their goodbyes. Rachel stops in briefly to say hello to their mom and then excuses herself to pick up her daughter at chorus. It's better to just let Leah visit by herself; besides, she's had enough for one day.

During the next two weeks Ruth has another difficult few days with a urinary tract infection and increased confusion. The nurse practitioner calls Rachel to discuss the situation and her care. After hearing the various options, Rachel decides that it's time to talk with someone from hospice. Rachel calls Leah to let her know that there is going to be an informational meeting with a hospice social worker on Friday, and hopefully, she can attend.

Rachel calmly explains to Leah, "Mom has lost ten more pounds in the past three months. She can't eat like she used to, and she is sleeping off and on throughout the day. Leah, we should be thinking about getting more end-of-life care and support."

"No, Rachel, I do not think that's what we or Mom needs right now! I can't believe you are just 'writing her off.' I am going to hang up now."

On Friday, Rachel and Ruth meet with the social worker, Pat, and registered nurse, Charlene, to learn about hospice and the additional expertise they can offer for end-of-life comfort measures. Pat explains that besides additional direct care staff, hospice will provide supplies, medications, emotional and spiritual support, and bereavement counseling for the family after Ruth dies. Charlene describes the trajectory of illness with dementia, the cascade of events that typically happens, and what that means for Ruth's prognosis. She also feels, along with the doctor, that Ruth is most likely in the final six months of her life. With tears in her eyes and a sigh of relief, Rachel tells them, "This is exactly what we need right now." They review which services Rachel wants for her mom, then she signs the paperwork to begin hospice care.

Rachel calls Leah to tell her about what she's learned and that hospice care is starting. Leah is at first silent, and then yells into the phone, "I can't believe you are doing this! Do you even care what I think?" and then hangs up. The next day, the social worker, Pat, reaches out to Leah, but she declines to meet with her.

One afternoon when Rachel comes to visit her mom, she sees her sitting in her wheelchair in the dining room. Her small frame is hunched over; her hands are tightly grasping the arms of the wheelchair, and her breathing is rapid. To Rachel, she clearly looks like she's in distress. She walks briskly back to the desk, where she sees the nurse standing in front of the medicine cart. "Hi, Tori, can you please give my mother some morphine for pain? She looks terribly uncomfortable sitting in the dining room."

Tori explains, "If we give her medicine for pain, though, she'll be too tired to eat."

Rachel feels the blood rise to her face and with measured speech says, "If she is in pain, she won't want to eat either! Would you please give her some pain medication and then return her to bed where she can rest and be more comfortable for now? I will offer her something to eat and drink once she feels better."

"Sure, I'll be in, in just a minute."

Rachel thanks her and walks back to the dining room. Just as Rachel is fixing the blanket over her mom's lap and getting ready to move her into her own room, Charlene from hospice arrives. Rachel catches Charlene's eye and shakes her head side to side. Charlene greets Ruth and then they walk in silence back to Ruth's bedroom. Rachel reiterates what just happened and vents to Charlene about all the stress she is under looking after her mom's care, dealing with her sister, and the stress at work.

Tori comes in with an aide and they assist Ruth back to bed. She gives her some liquid morphine under her tongue and covers her up with her red fleece blanket. Tori gives Charlene a quick update on Ruth's condition before returning to give her suppertime meds.

Charlene knows that the nursing home staff have tough jobs. They are often short-staffed and have large numbers of patients to care for. Charlene has been a hospice nurse for twenty years and has been visiting patients at Maple Village for most of that time. She knows that the team from hospice, the nursing home staff, and the family all have to work together, but sometimes that can be a challenge. She knows that it often takes sharing knowledge and talking things out.

Rachel and Charlene sit together, talking softly, as the late afternoon sun casts shadows around Ruth's room. Charlene peeks up at the bed and sees Ruth sleeping soundly and looking more relaxed. She offers to speak with the staff about putting Ruth back to bed when she doesn't look comfortable in her wheelchair, regardless of what time it is. Rachel readily accepts.

When Charlene walks behind the main desk of the unit, she is calm and engaging. She scans Ruth's chart and then begins to speak with Tori and two aides that are gathered at the desk. "Ruth seems to be having a tough time lately. I want to leave this chart that lists nonverbal signs of pain here with you.[3] At this point, it's better if she gets regularly scheduled pain medicine before bathing and moving around too much."[4] She explains to them the importance of comfort over "routine" and that when people are sick and nearing the end of their life, they often don't want to eat much. "It's a normal and natural process that happens at the end of life."

Tori and Charlene review Ruth's medication orders and Charlene writes a note on the clipboard to the nurse practitioner. Hospice offers to send a nurse out daily through the weekend to assure Rachel that her mom's pain is well managed. Charlene also arranges to send Ruth a hospice home health aide and volunteer to provide one-on-one personal care and presence.

Leah has now been visiting her mom every weekend. When it becomes clear that her mom is getting sicker and will not get better, Leah takes a family medical leave from work and visits the nursing home every day. She feels a mix of emotions from anxiety to sadness to anger. She continues to focus on what she can control: her mom's room and care.

One afternoon, Pat, the hospice social worker, comes by to visit Ruth. Pat tries to engage Leah by asking how her mom is doing, how she is doing, and what she can do to help. Leah barely makes eye contact. She keeps brushing her mom's hair away from her forehead and gives her a small amount of juice with a straw.

After a while, Leah begins to open up to Pat. "It's so hard for me to see my mom like this," she says. "She has always been bigger than life. I can't even imagine life without her. When my dad died, I felt like someone ripped my heart out. I had a very difficult time. He treated me like a princess. After this, it will just be me and Rachel. I'm worried about how that's going to go; I always feel so vulnerable around her. I already feel alone."

Pat just listens. Leah looks down at the floor and then out the window. After several minutes of silence, Leah begins to tell Pat stories about her mom: the time she brought a date home that her mom wasn't crazy about, the jewelry-making class they took together, and the summer vacation trips to the Catskills. At times, she wipes tears from her eyes, and at other times, she laughs as she retells some of her favorite memories. "I can't believe we've been sitting here for over an hour!" Leah gets up and gives Pat a big hug and thanks her for the visit.

Pat tells Leah how much she enjoyed talking with her. She reaches over and gently taps Ruth's shoulder. "Bye, Ruth. Rest well."

Before long, Ruth is no longer swallowing. She is bedbound and semiconscious. The spiritual counselor, Carole, visits often and reads psalms to Ruth from the Torah. Other hospice team members visit regularly and assist the nursing home staff in keeping Ruth comfortable and well cared for. One afternoon, as Ruth lay sleeping in her bed, both Rachel and Leah are sitting quietly at her bedside. The hospice harp player, Barbara, arrives and offers to play the harp for them. As the sweet music begins, tears stream down their cheeks. It is a special moment when the three of them can be together in peace. Right then, they know that in spite of all the stress and sadness, they will all be okay.

## REFLECTIONS ON RUTH AND FAMILY

Family relationships are complicated. When you add the stress of a sick or dying loved one, it can exacerbate family discord. Many family members are estranged from each other. Sometimes there's reconciliation and sometimes there's not. The good thing is, it's not hard to find common goals that everyone can get behind when someone is dying, such as: comfort, freedom from pain, and a peaceful death. Despite difficult past relationships, I have found that families often come together to care for each other.

Dementia can be particularly heart-wrenching. Ruth's behavior and communication was often unpredictable and foreign to her family. Rachel, as the decision-maker, had to guess sometimes what was going on with her mom and decide what to do. The approach to caring for someone with dementia has changed over time. Rather than constantly reorienting someone to the current situation, now the best approach is to allow the person to be wherever they are, and not try to make them be in "our world."[5] This can be really hard, especially when family members want the person to remember them and be "more normal." How we approach someone with dementia and what expectations we have can make a big difference in how we experience this relationship.[6] Try to look at people in the deepest possible way. People have tremendous value because of who they are, not because of how they look now, how they interact, or what they can't do anymore.

CHAPTER 7

# The Family Circle at the End of Life

"Manny! Manny!" Luis yells up to his nephew, accentuating the "Man" and letting the "ny" trail off. Footsteps come barreling down the stairs.

"What, Papi?" Manny's bulky frame fills the bedroom doorway.

"Go to the kitchen cabinet and grab my medicine bottles so the nurse here"—he nods toward Charlene—"can see what needs to be refilled." Luis directs Manny in Spanish. Sonia, the hospice interpreter, translates for Charlene. As Manny heads to the kitchen, Luis yells after him.

"I have the breathing machine medicine and sleeping pills here."

Hugging the blanket to his chest, Luis turns on his side and opens the bedside table drawer. "I have two boxes of the nebulizer medicine, but I need some more sleeping pills." He holds up the bottle to show Charlene.

Manny returns with a red plastic basket filled with pill bottles and hands it over to Luis. Charlene picks up each pill bottle and the inhaler box from the basket and checks how much medicine is left.

With each container, Luis answers a series of questions as Sonia interprets, "What is your pain level? Are you taking much breakthrough pain medicine? How's your breathing?

Are you moving your bowels?" Charlene takes notes in her spiral notebook as Luis, Manny, and Sonia fire away rapidly in Spanish. They finish up their visit and let Luis know they'll be back again in a couple of days.

Luis is 5 foot, 4 inches tall, strong as an ox, and commander of his own ship. He worked hard all his life at various docks along the eastern seaboard, loading and unloading cargo containers.

He moved around a lot and made many friends over the course of his life. He once told Sonia that he made some enemies too. "And I have the scars to prove it!"

Luis moved to the mainland US from Puerto Rico when he was in his early twenties. He still has several siblings and cousins who live on the island. Once Luis retired, he moved into an apartment near his sister, Yarelis, and her family. Luis meticulously managed every aspect of his life. He bought his own food, cooked his own meals, took care of his apartment and his truck, and managed his medical problems. "I kept track of everything—when filters needed to be changed, tires needed rotating, and medicines needed refills." For years, Luis was seeing his doctors to manage his diabetes, emphysema, prostate problems, and bad knees. He kept his appointments, took his medicine, and mostly followed his diet.

Just after turning seventy-three, Luis began to feel winded whenever he walked up the stairs to his apartment. He found himself using his inhaler more often and it didn't seem to help much anymore. His coughing fits got longer and more frequent until he started coughing up pink phlegm. After a series of tests, his doctor confirmed that Luis had advanced lung cancer. He was offered chemotherapy. "I knew things were bad," he recalled. "I would go through a lot without it giving me any more time. I saw my cousin go through the same thing. No, gracias."

Because of the cancer, Luis had a large accumulation of fluid between his chest wall and his lungs. He underwent a procedure to place a tube into this space to drain the fluid out. That's when his doctor arranged to have regular visits by a nurse who would attach a vacuum container to the tube and drain out the fluid to help his breathing.

That's also when his sister, Yarelis, told him it was time for him to move in with her. "I didn't want to leave my apartment, but I knew I had to, especially with this tube." Yarelis and her son, Manny, set up a room for Luis just off the front hall. The bedroom is very small, but everything is in close reach. There's only a narrow path between the walls and the hospital bed on both sides. A bedside table is positioned on the left side of the bed, where a nebulizer machine and hoses cover the top surface. A large oxygen machine rests against the wall on the right side of the room. The wall at the end of the hospital bed holds a makeshift closet and a tall dresser with a television on top, tuned to a Spanish language talk show. The walls have thin brown paneling and a low ceiling of white wainscoting. When Manny's kids and dogs are over, Luis can hear everything.

Outside, the dogs start barking loudly and jumping up and down, causing the chain-link fence to clink repeatedly. The kids are screeching in the backyard as the doorbell rings in the front. Luis hears Yarelis answer the door and greet Charlene and Sonia again.

"Hola!" Sonia says as she steps into the front hall.

"Oh my goodness, it smells amazing in here!" Charlene says as she lifts up her head and inhales deeply through her nose.

"I'm cooking some pork adobo with rice and beans. I hope Luis can eat some."

Yarelis leads Charlene and Sonia into Luis's room, where he's already setting up the supplies to drain the fluid.

Luis gathers up his glasses, cell phone, television remote, and tissue box, and moves them out of the way as he guardedly turns onto his left side. Charlene starts by listening to Luis's lungs and abdomen and checking his blood pressure, pulse, and temperature. She then sets up a sterile drape on the bed and gently removes the old bandage from the right side of his chest, revealing a tube coiled into a circle and capped. She uncaps the tube, straightens it out, releases the clamps, and attaches the vacuum container to the tube. Immediately a pale yellow fluid sprays into the bottle.

"How are you doing, Luis?" Sonia asks, peeking over to check on him.

Luis takes a deep breath, nods, and says, "Better," as the fluid finally slows to a drip. "It's such a relief to have this fluid taken out."

Charlene disconnects the bottle, clamps and caps the tube, and applies a fresh bandage to his chest. "Okay, my friend," Charlene says as Luis slowly turns over onto his back.

Sonia and Luis go on to talk about his family, what he's been eating, and how he's managing. She learns that Luis's sister, Yarelis, attends church or a prayer group every day. Luis hasn't been active in any church or religion for years. He declines visits by the hospice chaplain, social worker, and aide. "Manny helps me in the shower. I don't need anybody," Luis says as he waves his hand away.

Sonia and Charlene finish up their visit and encourage Luis to call if he's uncomfortable or if he has any complications.

They each shake his hand, cover the handshake with their left hand, and warmly say, "Adiós."

As Charlene and Sonia open the gate and head to their separate cars, Charlene says, "Luis is a man of few words, but he certainly knows what he wants!"

"No kidding," Sonia agrees, smiling and shaking her head. "His strength and will are remarkable."

Over the next several weeks, Luis gets weaker and needs more help getting around. Manny helps him transfer into the wheelchair so he can sit out in the living room in the recliner for an hour every afternoon. He now relies on the oxygen when he moves around during the day and all through the night. His appetite has also waned quite a bit. He still likes his coffee, farina, and his sister's chicken soup, but anything heavier just doesn't taste that good anymore.

Yarelis tells Sonia that she's worried about Luis not eating. She explains in detail what he's had to eat so far that day and how it is less than usual. "His cheeks look so thin and his eyes are so dark," Yarelis says, shaking her head and putting her hand on her chest. Sonia tries to explain that this is what normally happens when someone is so sick. She tells Yarelis that she knows how hard this is as she reaches over and gives her a hug.

Luis always wears a loose pullover sweatshirt and flannel pajama bottoms; his weight loss isn't as obvious on his small frame. His voice is hoarser, but he still runs the show: "Manny, get me my inhaler; don't forget my glasses; bring me some water."

One day Charlene and Sonia arrive for their biweekly visit. Yarelis greets them at the door and, speaking hurriedly in Spanish, tells Sonia that Luis isn't good today. "He's restless and can't breathe."

Luis is sitting upright in bed, his oxygen tube is in his nose, and he's repeatedly coughing into a tissue. His chest is rising up and down as he tries to cough up phlegm. Luis's face is moist and his eyes are open wide as he looks up at Charlene and Sonia and shakes his head. Charlene immediately checks his condition and finds that he has a temperature of 101.6 degrees, his blood pressure and pulse are elevated, and his lungs are congested. She checks his oxygen level, gives him a breathing treatment with the nebulizer, and administers acetaminophen for his fever as well as morphine and lorazepam to ease his breathing.[1] Charlene encourages Luis to put a pillow up against his chest, and to hug the pillow as he tries to get a stronger cough. Charlene contacts the hospice doctor, who suspects that Luis has a respiratory infection and makes arrangements for a liquid antibiotic prescription to be sent to his pharmacy.

When Charlene goes into the living room to gather the supplies she needs to drain the fluid from Luis's chest, she notices that every seat in the living room is now full of older women sitting quietly with their hands folded in their laps. She also hears three to four voices coming from the kitchen, all speaking in Spanish. Charlene greets them by nodding hello and asks Sonia to explain to Yarelis and the others what appears to be going on with Luis. Most of the women are from the church. They join Yarelis in a circle to offer prayers for Luis.

Sonia gives instructions to Manny, who gathers his keys and phone and rushes out to pick up the new medicine for Luis. Charlene finishes up her treatments and says goodbye, reminding Luis and Yarelis to call her if he's in distress: "Please don't wait until my regular visits to let me know that you don't feel well." Charlene and Sonia walk out together. They open the front gate and, before parting ways, talk briefly about how much they wish families would call hospice right away when something is wrong.

Over the next several days, Luis's breathing is better, but he continues to get weaker and eats less and less. He no longer goes out into the living room to sit every afternoon. He mostly stays in bed and is sleeping more and more. At one visit, Charlene learns that Luis is bothered by constipation; at another visit, he is experiencing anxiety on and off during the night. Charlene talks with Luis and his family, and then makes recommendations to alleviate the problems that come up.

During one visit, Yarelis whispers to Sonia in the living room, "I think Luis is afraid of dying and that's why he's not sleeping that good at night."

"I'm sure it's hard. He's been so strong. Charlene and I will talk with him and see if he'll open up a bit. We can also offer a social work visit, but so far, he hasn't been interested in visits from other team members."

"Luis, we know this is all really hard," Sonia begins as she sits next to him on the bed. "You've been incredibly strong. It's normal to worry about how things are going to go. A lot of people do."

Luis looks down and moves the tissue around in his hand but doesn't say anything.

After a few seconds, Sonia continues. "We're going to take good care of you, along with your family, Luis. We'll also help manage any symptoms that might come up."

Luis looks up at Sonia and then over at Charlene and nods slightly.

"Do you want to talk with our social worker or chaplain, Luis?" Sonia asks tentatively. "They help people a lot, and they're really easy to talk to."

Before Sonia can explain what they do, Luis shakes his head and waves his hand. He pulls his blanket up to his chest and looks up at the television.

Charlene and Sonia glance at each other briefly. Charlene gets up and takes stock of what supplies and medicines Luis needs. Sonia sits quietly next to Luis as he slowly drifts off to sleep.

Over the next week, Luis is sleeping all the time. He hasn't had anything to eat at all. He's getting mouth care with moist swabs and lip balm. His breathing has become shallow, but it's not labored, and he seems calm and peaceful.

One late afternoon, Yarelis calls the office sobbing and tells hospice that Luis has just died. Several family members were in his room talking to him, holding his hand and praying. His breathing slowed down and just stopped. Yarelis tearfully tells Sonia that she had just left his room and was in the kitchen when her niece cried out to let everyone know that he had just died.

When Sonia and Charlene arrive, the house is full. Family members fill the kitchen and living room, talking and crying and hugging each other. They take turns going into Luis's room, since only a few people can fit in the small pathways around his bed. Several people clear out, leaving room for Charlene and Sonia to make the pronouncement that Luis has indeed died. Charlene gently removes the oxygen tubing from Luis's nose and reaches over to turn the machine off. The room becomes silent as Luis's small body lies still in the large hospital bed.

With the help of Manny and his cousin, they wash, dress, and position Luis's body slightly upright in his bed. A navy blue fleece blanket covers his lower body and his hands are folded in his lap. After Sonia and Charlene finish and gather up their supplies, they invite others to come back into the room. They thank everyone for taking such good care of Luis.

For the last time, Sonia and Charlene part ways by the gate and hug each other.

"What an amazing spirit Luis had," Sonia reflects.

"I know," Charlene agrees. "And a beautiful, loving family too."

## REFLECTIONS ON LUIS AND FAMILY

People who are faced with adversity often have an extraordinary amount of strength. Even the smallest, sickest person, like Luis, can demonstrate an incredible amount of toughness and courage. It's important to give people as much control over their own care as they want. Being in control of one's own decisions can reduce feelings of powerlessness and frustration and can improve a person's sense of independence and well-being.[2] Sometimes family members, visitors, and health care people talk *about* someone, rather than *to* them. As someone's disease gets worse, it can be hard for family members to know when to speak for someone and when to let them handle things themself. Try to address the person who is sick first. It establishes a respect for their presence and point of view. Family members and others can then fill in the rest of the story as needed.

Caring for a loved one who is dying should be more of a family event than a medical one. Families share an incredible richness and history. Everyone has a unique relationship to each other and to the person who is dying.

Culture, language, and religion are central to many families.[3] During major milestones of a family's life, such as births, weddings, and deaths, the culture of a family is also celebrated. Luis was cared for by his sister, nephew, and extended family; this was accepted in his culture. Many families have an identified "primary caregiver," but some families don't. They struggle to provide care around the clock. Hospice can help families arrange for more care, if needed. Caring for a person who is sick and dying can be physically and emotionally draining. There is often intense sadness and fatigue. It can also be a time of profound gratitude and togetherness. The care provided by family members to each other is a blessing that I am forever grateful to witness.

CHAPTER 8

# Dealing with the Crisis of Pain

"I don't know what to do. He's in terrible pain. Maybe he should have stayed at the hospital," Alison says with tears in her eyes as she greets the hospice nurse at the door. "I tried to call the doctor at the hospital, but I can't get through. The ambulance dropped him off about an hour ago. I've been running around all morning, trying to move things around and clear out a room for him." Alison talks rapidly as she directs Charlene through her kitchen and into the hallway. Alison's long brown hair is gathered up in an elastic on the top of her head, with strands loosely falling out here and there. Her oversize red hooded sweatshirt hangs loose on her small frame. The sleeves extend beyond her hands, which she keeps up by her face, alternating covering her mouth and wiping her eyes. She leads Charlene to a small room off the hall and extends her hand as a way of introduction to her father, Ray.

Ray is lying face down, diagonally, on a twin-size hospital bed. His legs are drawn up as he holds his stomach and moans. He still has his baseball cap, tan work boots, and hospital bracelet on.

"Ray, my name is Charlene. I'm a nurse, and I'm going to help you as soon as possible."

Charlene directs Alison to get the packet with his hospital discharge paperwork.

"He said they gave him some pain medicine before he left the hospital," Alison reports as she passes a blue plastic folder to Charlene.

Kneeling down next to Ray, Charlene shuffles through a large stack of papers until she finds a sheet highlighted and labeled "Discharge Instructions." She quickly scans the instructions until she finds the discharge medication list. She sees that four prescriptions were sent over to the local pharmacy. Unfortunately, none of them are a long-acting pain medication.

"I'm sorry," Alison says as she stands over her dad and Charlene, wiping her eyes with her sleeve. "I haven't had two seconds to run to the pharmacy."

"It's okay, Alison. These things happen. But your dad needs medicine right away. I'm going to call his doctor and ask for another prescription to be sent over to the pharmacy immediately. Is there anyone who can pick these up now?"

"No, it's just me. My brother lives in Florida, and everybody else I could ask is working."

Charlene offers to stay with Ray while Alison runs to the pharmacy. She immediately gets on the phone and asks Ray's doctor to consider ordering a long-acting pain medicine in addition to the other prescriptions. She also tells the doctor's office that she will call the doctor back and give a full report on his condition once he's settled. Charlene also calls the hospice office and asks if one of the social workers is available to come over this afternoon.

Ray turns onto his side. His knees are drawn up and he is wincing in pain, and his face is flushed. Charlene grabs a cold pack from the freezer and tucks it up against his belly, hoping that it might distract him from the pain, if nothing else. She grabs a pillow and puts it up against his stomach and encourages him to hug the pillow and try to focus on his breathing. She demonstrates, counting three breaths, in and out. She rubs his back gently as he tries to follow her instructions.

While Charlene waits for Alison to return, she grabs a blue desk chair, rolls it over next to Ray's bed, and sits down. She looks around the room. Pushed to the opposite wall is a large desk with a laptop and what looks like stacks of papers and catalogs. A calendar on the wall has a picture of a skier on a mountain of snow wearing colorful gear against a bright blue sky. Several sticky notes hang from the calendar and on the wall.

Charlene looks at the discharge paperwork again. She reads: *Raymond Benson. Age 64. Diagnosis: Colon cancer, stage IV, distant lymph nodes enlarged, hypertension, hypercholesteremia. Underwent a limited sigmoidoscopy and biopsy. Declined further testing and evaluation.*

"Doing okay, Ray?" Charlene asks. Getting no response, she reaches over, rubs his shoulder, and says, "Alison should be back shortly. The medicine will help pretty quickly."

She continues reading: *Not a candidate for surgery. Probable liver mass and lymph node involvement. Declined short-term rehab. Plan: Discharge to daughter's home. Referral to VNA (Visiting Nurse Association).* Charlene shakes her head. Thankfully her agency's liaison to the hospital intercepted this referral and suggested that a hospice nurse go out first and evaluate him. A referral to the VNA rather than hospice would have meant that Ray was electing a rehabilitation approach to his care, which he had declined.

Charlene hears the kitchen door open and Alison yell, "I'm back."

Alison comes into the bedroom and passes the bag to Charlene. "Sorry it took so long; they had to fill the new one while I was there. Let me go get some water. Dad, you okay?" she yells back as she heads out of the room.

Charlene gives Ray a dose of the short-acting pain medicine. "This will take several minutes to kick in, Ray, but you will feel better shortly. I'm going to go out into the kitchen and talk with Alison a bit, but I'll come back in to check on you. I'll wait until you're feeling a bit better before I complete my full assessment." Ray looks up and nods slightly. Alison and Charlene head back down the hallway and settle into chairs in the small kitchen.

"Let's chat for a few minutes," Charlene begins, "until your dad is feeling better."

Alison reaches her arms up and puts both elbows on the table, resting her head in her hands. "I'm not sure what to do. A few days ago, I got a call from the doctor telling me that my father is in the hospital. He said he has colon cancer that has probably spread. I had not seen my father for at least three months! Yesterday, the case manager calls and says he refuses to go to rehab; we need to discharge him tomorrow. I could not believe what I was hearing. He can't take care of himself. I wasn't sure what else to do, so I had him come here."

"Well. I'm sorry about all this, Alison, but we'll help you sort this all out. One of our social workers is free to come over shortly, if that's okay with you. She will help you arrange for more care. We're also here to help you, Alison," Charlene reassures her.

"Well, I need all the help I can get," Alison says emphatically. "Can I get you something to drink?" After Charlene declines, Alison gets up and pours herself some coffee.

Charlene gets right down to business. She clarifies that even though the hospital had initially made a referral for home nursing and rehab, Ray's wishes are more in line with hospice: no more tests, hospitals, and chemotherapy.

"That's what he said at the hospital meeting," Alison confirms. "Oh my God, was that only yesterday? It feels like a week ago!"

"I know, there's a lot going on. Why don't we go over some details for a few minutes until our social worker, Pat, arrives, then I'll go back in and check on him."

Charlene reviews with Alison what additional equipment might be helpful and then suggests a commode, urinal, wheelchair, and bath bench for Ray. She also reviews the medications that are prescribed and the schedule. Charlene writes down the instructions and makes it clear not to skip any doses. "It's very important that he receives this long-acting pain pill every twelve hours, on schedule." She also reviews other important information, such as what he can eat, the importance of preventing falls, and to call hospice anytime, day or night, if needed.

While Charlene follows up and makes a few calls in the kitchen, Alison heads back to see how her dad is doing. "Dad, has the pain let up?"

Ray turns his head and looks up at Alison. "A little bit. The pill definitely took the edge off."

She immediately notices that his eyes look brighter and more relaxed. Just as she is about to relay the information that she and Charlene just talked about, they hear someone else come in. "Hang on a second, Dad."

"Alison, this is our social worker, Pat," Charlene says. "I thought maybe the two of you could chat while I check on your dad. How's he doing?"

"A little better," she says. "I was just going to see if he wants anything."

Charlene and Alison catch Pat up a bit on the situation and the plan so far. They all go back in and greet Ray and share some details with him as well. They discuss how he's doing and then Charlene sits down with him to complete her assessment.

Alison and Pat head back to the kitchen. Alison's not exactly sure what a hospice social worker does, so she is relieved when Pat explains, "I'm here to support you and your family emotionally, and to help secure additional services for you, if you want."

Alison takes a deep breath. "Well, I'm not sure where to begin," she says as so many thoughts come rushing into her head.

"Let's start by telling me about your family," Pat suggests. "Are there other people available to help and support you?"

"I have one brother, Bill, who lives in Florida. It's just us. Plus I have a lot of support from my friends and neighbors."

Alison looks over at Pat. She has bright blue eyes and soft white hair. Alison instantly feels comfortable talking with Pat, like she is talking with a friend over coffee. Pat jots a few notes down in her a notebook as Alison shares her family story. "It's complicated," she begins.

Alison tells Pat that when she was in middle school, her parents got divorced. Her dad's drinking played a big role in her parents' divorce, as there were many nights of fighting leading up to the separation and divorce. Alison, Bill, who's three years older, and their mother, Joan, had a tough time emotionally and financially after the divorce. Soon after graduation from high school, Bill moved to Florida, started up a business, and settled there with his family. Alison went to a local community college to study fashion merchandising then went on to the local university for her college degree. Just two months after graduating from college, Alison's mother, Joan, died suddenly of a brain aneurism.

"I was devastated; my mother and I were very close. I was a mess. She was my biggest cheerleader in life. She was the one who helped me finish school and land my first job as a buyer for a well-known clothing store."

"I'm so sorry, Alison. That's so traumatic."

"It was awful," Alison goes on. "Thank God for my friends. Between them, a therapist, and a bereavement group, I was able to move on and face my new life without her."

"I can certainly understand how hard this must be for you now," Pat offers.

"It is. I only saw my father every few months, usually when he needed my help with something," Alison continues. "Over the years, he worked off and on at various car sales and car repair businesses. He became disabled after an injury at work; he worked in the service department of a local car repair business. I always wondered if his drinking played a role in the accident, although no one ever mentioned that, at least not to me. My father continued to drink, especially after that."

Alison takes a sip of her coffee and continues. "He also had a number of girlfriends over the years. None of them seemed to have any interest in getting to know me or my brother, though. I feel like our relationship has been complicated and distant. You know, I blame him for many of my family's problems, but I also love him and feel sorry for him. It also bothers me, on some level, that my mother died so young while my father took such poor care of himself and is still alive," Alison admits, surprised that she is sharing all this.

"He's my father, though. I didn't know what else to do. He's not about to move to Florida," she says with her hands outstretched.

Pat reassures Alison that hospice will help her secure more care, but if this doesn't work out, then they will help to arrange care for him elsewhere.

"Well, we'll see," Alison says. "The good thing is, everyone at work has been amazing. I have this whole week off, and then I can apply for a family leave if I have to. My friends have also been great. They're all willing to help, and my neighbors have already offered to do whatever I need. I'm fortunate there."

Charlene comes into the kitchen as Pat and Alison are just finishing up. "He's doing better; he's dozing off," Charlene reports. She reviews the handwritten instructions again.

Alison nods in agreement and puts the instructions on her refrigerator. "Thank you both so much," she says as they say their goodbyes and hug.

"I'll be back tomorrow with Luz, one of our home health aides," Charlene says. "In the meantime, please call us with any questions whatsoever."

Charlene and Pat head out together. They chat briefly before going their separate ways. They agree that it's so frustrating when families are so often put in this situation: discharged home with unmanaged symptoms, lots of stress, and so many loose ends to tie up. "I just feel so bad for them both," Pat says as she heads to her car.

The following day, Charlene arrives with Luz, the aide. When they come into the kitchen, they are surprised to see Ray sitting up at the kitchen table having coffee and a piece of toast! Alison reports that she stuck to the pain medicine schedule and her dad slept all night. "Good thing he had the urinal too; he didn't even have to find his way to the bathroom."

"That's great," Charlene says. "Yesterday was a rough day; I'm so glad you're better, Ray." She reintroduces herself to Ray, and introduces Luz.

After breakfast, Luz helps Ray wash up and get dressed. Charlene and Alison review the medication chart that Alison filled in. They also review the health care proxy and the DNR form. Ray made it clear that he doesn't want any more treatments, including no resuscitation or hospitals. "Call us first," Charlene reminds them.

Charlene reviews with Alison what to expect in the upcoming weeks, such as a decrease in her dad's appetite, more fatigue, and more time spent sleeping.[1] She also talks about the importance of pain medication, not waiting until the pain gets worse before taking a short-acting pill, and about preventing constipation and nausea.[2]

They hear Luz walking with Ray back into his bedroom, so they both head there. "He's a new man!" Luz proclaims as she passes him a hairbrush and gathers up her supplies.

"He sure is," Charlene agrees. She pulls up a chair and begins to ask Ray a series of questions about how he feels and what else he might want.

*There's a lot of history to untangle here*, Alison thinks as she looks over at her father sitting at the edge of the bed in his white T-shirt and Dickies. She notices bruises on the top of his hands and on the inside of his elbows that she didn't see yesterday. She watches him interact with Charlene and Luz. His answers sound a bit short and gruff, but soon he seems to warm up to them and even jokes with them a little. He shrugs but agrees to have a hospice volunteer and spiritual counselor come out and visit with him. For once, she feels a glimmer of hope that maybe this will work out, and it might even be good for him—and for her too.

Pat comes back out that afternoon. She talks with Ray and Alison about additional community services that might be helpful, such as an emergency button, meals-on-wheels, and a hospice respite, if needed. They also start to talk openly about the emotional burdens of their relationship, their losses, and their hopes going forward.

As the weeks go on, the hospice team visits Ray and Alison every few days and helps them understand what is going on and how to manage his care. Alison's friends and neighbors bring over food and stay with her dad so she can get out. Alison's brother, Bill, comes up from Florida to visit his dad and to give Alison a break. Alison and Bill really enjoy this time together. They reconnect, and they talk a lot about their parents, their life, and their future. It's all a whirlwind, but both Alison and Ray now have hope that they can handle what's next with the help of each other and from hospice.

## REFLECTIONS ON RAY AND FAMILY

Ray and Alison's scenario is so common and so stressful. So much of end-of-life care is about having the knowledge of what to expect in the final months, weeks, and days of life. It also requires having information about symptoms, medications, and personal care needs. This is all happening at a time of intense emotion, confusion, and fatigue. How can anyone deal with any of this when they are in pain or if they're watching their loved one in so much pain? It's excruciating.

Symptom management is key to a family's quality of life when someone is at the end of life. Not everyone experiences symptoms, but cancer and other diseases often cause distress. Common symptoms that people experience are: pain, difficulty breathing, anxiety, fatigue, confusion, nausea, vomiting, and constipation.[3] Hospice will recommend both medications and non-medication treatments to relieve whatever symptoms come up.

Since hospice staff aren't with the person who is dying all the time, families often find themselves in the position of having to interpret what symptoms are occurring with their loved one, deciding whether they should give a medicine or not, and if so, how much. It can be an overwhelming and scary position to be in. Hospice team members want families to contact them whenever any symptoms arise or if they have any questions. The relief of pain and other symptoms is one of the most important benefits of hospice care.[4] Hospice educates and supports families day-to-day, and they help manage any symptoms that might come up. How the end-of-life process goes, and how comfortable the dying person is during this time, can affect family members positively or negatively during their bereavement process.[5]

It's hard for families like Ray's to know what care options are available when a loved one is sick. The eligibility and availability of various programs are hard to understand, especially when family members are dealing with a loved one who is seriously ill and having a medical crisis. It's helpful for families to understand beforehand what the differences are between traditional care and comfort care, and between palliative care and hospice care.[6] For anyone who has been diagnosed with a serious or terminal illness, a palliative care consult or a hospice informational visit can provide this information.

Unfortunately, admission to hospice care often feels like an emergency situation. Sometimes this happens because people are discharged home from the hospital somewhat abruptly after curative care stops working, or, like Ray, they choose not to have any further testing. In some cases, people are at home and their condition worsens. Instead of calling 911 and going to the hospital, they decide that they "just can't go back there again." Their doctor then recommends hospice instead. Hospice often walks into an emergency room–like situation. This is so stressful for families. They are trying to understand what is going on medically, what is recommended, and how everything works. They are also communicating with hospital personnel, hospice staff, delivery people, and sometimes nursing home staff. The amount of communication and coordination needed to set up care at home is tremendous. Families should take any opportunity they can to learn more about how the system works and options for medical care, especially when someone has a serious illness like cancer, heart disease, or lung disease.

CHAPTER 9

# Morphine Doesn't Kill People, Diseases Do

Roger is a construction worker who is "tough as nails." He's a guy who can fix anything, will lend a helping hand, or give you the shirt off his back. He has worked hard all his life. Roger began smoking when he was only fourteen years old and has kept up a two-packs-a-day habit for at least fifty years. Roger had a hacking morning cough most of the time, but when he reached sixty years old, he started to get winded after exerting himself. He made adjustments, slowed down, and then officially retired at age sixty-five. He continues to do odd jobs for a number of people, works on various projects in his garage, and spends more time with his six adult children and a growing number of grandchildren.

Roger's family adores him. His wife and children always fuss over him; he waves off this attention, but with pride. His wife, Lorraine, can usually be found in the kitchen, whipping up meat pies or French pastries. She wears bright, colorful blouses with flowers and greets everyone with a cheerful "Hello, so nice to see you!" She is a devout Catholic who goes to church every Sunday. She is also on a number of committees at the church and enjoys church socials, especially weekly bingo and the annual church picnic. Roger goes to the annual picnic and the special masses, like Christmas and Easter, but he doesn't really care to get all dolled up for church each week, nor does he have any interest in regular social events. What he does like to do is go to tag sales every Saturday with Lorraine. He occasionally picks up a tool, but mostly he enjoys strolling by the various vendors and checking out the goods.

One morning Roger is in his garage working under the hood of his truck. Lorraine comes to the doorway, drying her hands on her apron. Looking alarmed, she says, "Roger, there's blood in the toilet! What's going on? Should we get that checked out?"

He peers up from under the hood. "My throat's just a bit sore. Nothing to worry about."

About a week later, Roger gets up and sits on the side of the bed. Sweat is dripping off of him and his breathing is labored. Alarmed, Lorraine calls the ambulance to take Roger to the hospital.

After a week of doctors, blood tests, X-rays, and scans, Roger is diagnosed with pneumonia, COPD (chronic obstructive pulmonary disease), and lung cancer. His family is shocked and scared. Roger was always strong; now he is in a hospital bed with oxygen on and IV lines going into his chest and arms, and he's drifting in and out of wakefulness. His family takes turns coming in to visit. Lorraine spends hours at his bedside praying, encouraging him, and helping the nurses care for him. Everyone keeps telling Lorraine to "go home, take a nap, get something to eat, and take care of yourself." Lorraine keeps telling them that she is fine, she never naps, and she has been eating. The hospital kitchen has sent her a tray of food every lunchtime since Roger was admitted.

After three to four days, Roger seems to "come out of it." He is more alert, taking sips of water and answering short questions correctly. By the end of the week, he is sitting up in a chair, eating soft foods, and visiting with his family. His pneumonia is clearing. The doctors and social worker ask for a family meeting to discuss the medical plan going forward. Roger just keeps insisting that he go home.

Lorraine sits in Roger's hospital room watching the lab technician set up the supplies to draw blood from Roger's arm.

"Do I have any blood left?" Roger asks jokingly.

Just then, Bob, Roger and Lorraine's oldest son, enters the room. "Well, it sounds like you're feeling better," he says as he walks past the end of the bed, squeezes his dad's toes, and bends down and kisses his mom on the cheek. "How are you doing, Dad?"

"I'm fine, and I'll be better as soon as I get out of here!"

"Well, then, let's hope that's the plan."

Lorraine catches Bob up on the medical staff who have come in so far that morning and what's been said. "A kidney doctor came in earlier to see him, and that's why he's having more blood tests. The lung doctor is pleased that his breathing is better; he's starting him on a new inhaler. He said when he does go home, they'll switch him over to an antibiotic pill instead of the bag." She points up to a bag on an IV pole over the bed.

"Any word on when that will be?" Bob asks, looking at his mother then his father.

Just then, two women arrive in the doorway and knock. The woman with the white coat and long dark hair introduces herself as Dr. Patel, an oncologist. She introduces Mary, a social worker, from the Cancer Center. After initial introductions, they all sit around Roger's bed and discuss the status of his cancer.

It's hard for Roger to pay attention to any of these details. For one thing, he can't hear very well, and for another thing, it sounds like they're speaking another language. He hears the doctor say "non-small cell" and "lymph nodes." She goes on to talk about treatment for this type of cancer, which is chemotherapy. He hears percentages: with treatment, without treatment, a new combination approach with targeted therapy, promising results . . .

Bob asks, "Could he have surgery and just remove the cancer? What would the schedule be for chemotherapy? Would he have to be in the hospital for that?" The doctor calmly answers all of his questions. Lorraine sits quietly with her hands folded in her lap.

Mary looks up at Roger and says, "Roger, are you understanding what the doctor is saying? Do you have any questions?"

"What I understand is that I don't want any of that; I just want to go home."

Mary smiles. "I hear what you're saying. Either way, it sounds like you'll be discharged today or tomorrow. But do you understand what the doctor is saying about the cancer and the treatment?"

"I know, I got cancer. What else is there to say?"

"Well, we just want to make sure that you have an opportunity to ask whatever questions you might have."

Bob and the doctor continue to discuss the test results, what findings are still pending, and the various options available. Finally Bob says, "Well, I think we need some time to let this all sink in."

"Of course," both Mary and Dr. Patel say in unison.

"We'll set you up with a discharge appointment in a week or two," the doctor adds. That will give you some time to get home, and hopefully get stronger."

"Sounds good," Bob says.

After Dr. Patel and Mary reiterate the plan and say their goodbyes, Roger looks over at Lorraine. “Well, honey?”

The truth is, both Lorraine and Bob know that Roger has no intention of getting more tests, needles, or chemotherapy. They can’t even picture it. He is one tough character, but not when it comes to medical things. He never even went to a doctor until he was at least fifty.

The following day, Roger signs a DNR form. Lorraine packs up his belongings and Roger is discharged home with a referral for hospice care.

That same afternoon, Charlene, the nurse, arrives and begins hospice services for Roger and his family. “Roger, one of the questions I ask all patients is, What are your goals? In other words, what is most important to you right now?”

Well, breathing, for one thing! That would be important! I don’t want to be gasping for air!” Roger exclaims from his favorite recliner in the family room. I also like going out to lunch with Lorraine on Saturdays, you know, and checking out some tag sales.”

“We can definitely help you with that.” Charlene smiles as she grabs her stethoscope and begins to listen to his lungs.

At home, Roger slowly gets stronger. Charlene encourages him to take small doses of liquid morphine before bed, first thing in the morning, and before any exertion. Roger is skeptical: “I don’t want to get addicted to this stuff, and besides, it will probably kill me before the cancer does!”[1]

Charlene smiles then explains, “Many people worry about that, Roger, but addiction is generally not a concern for people with cancer who use opioids, like morphine, to manage pain or difficulty breathing.[2] With the right dose, it is exactly what you need right now to meet your goal of breathing easier and getting out with Lorraine.”[3]

Sure enough, Roger follows the medication plan and feels much better and is going out again on his Saturday trips. His family visits more often now. Roger declines any additional help from the hospice team, such as a social worker or home health aide. "I can take care of myself."

After a few more weeks, though, Roger begins to wake up at night with difficulty breathing. The short-acting liquid medicine is only holding him for two hours, so he is waking up every two hours struggling to catch his breath. Charlene requests some oxygen, a fan, a bed wedge to keep his head elevated, and a long-acting version of morphine.[4] Immediately, Roger is sleeping through the night. "I don't want to take that stuff during the day, though, because it makes me feel too fuzzy," Roger says emphatically.

"That's fine," Charlene tells him. "You're driving this bus. You can just keep taking the short-acting liquid during the day when you need it."

Roger does fine again for another several weeks. He spends time with his family, putters around his garage, and continues to go out on Saturdays with Lorraine. He's not eating as much as he used to, but he's still eating three meals a day. Roger's holding his own.

By this time, it is late September, almost three months since Roger was hospitalized. The doctors said that without chemotherapy, his cancer would continue to grow. He would likely get more respiratory infections, and his prognosis is probably not more than three months. "What am I supposed to do, just lie down and die?" he says whenever anyone comments on his exceeding all expectations. He still refuses any personal care assistance and declines any social or spiritual help. "What am I supposed to talk about? It is what it is."

As the days get colder, Roger has a harder time getting out. He starts to hang on to the furniture and walls when he walks. He hasn't gone out of the house for three weeks now. Roger tells Charlene that he needs to take the short-acting liquid morphine every hour or two during the day now so he can breathe. He agrees to take the long-acting morphine both at night and during the day, and it helps. Hospice also delivers him a seat lift chair and a walker. The lift recliner helps him get out of his chair without rocking, but he declines to use the walker.

Soon enough, Roger is sleeping most of the day in his recliner. He transfers back and forth to his bed at night. He still insists on walking to the bathroom to wash up and toilet. "No one is going to wipe my ass," he insists.

Over the next two weeks, his family visits often. Roger consents to having the priest come over, mostly for Lorraine. He spends most of the time sleeping. He struggles to walk to the bathroom, but he insists. He declines a hospital bed, and he continues to resist any additional help from his family or hospice. Since he can't swallow pills anymore, Charlene starts a morphine infusion by putting a small needle in his belly. The small pump delivers a consistent amount of morphine around the clock. It keeps him comfortable and breathing easily.

Days later, on a Sunday morning, Lorraine and her daughter, Claire, leave for eleven o'clock mass and Bob comes over to stay with his dad. Roger is in his bed with his head elevated on pillows and oxygen tubing in his nose. His breathing is shallow and quiet and he's unresponsive. Bob goes into the kitchen to make himself a sandwich. When he comes back into the bedroom, he stops short when he realizes that his father isn't breathing. He has just died. Just then, Lorraine and Claire enter the house. Bob calls for them to come right in.

After the initial shock, they all sit quietly at Roger's bedside and say a prayer together.

They remember that Charlene told them that sometimes people "slip away" when no one is in the room. They reflect on their husband and father. They share stories, laugh, and marvel at his independence and strength of character. And no one ever "wiped his ass."

## REFLECTIONS ON ROGER AND FAMILY

I have found that people often go through the dying process the same way they live. If they are strong-willed, comical, analytical, and accepting, they often show these same qualities as they are dying. I often hear families say, "Well, she hasn't lost her sense of humor" or "He's a fighter to the end." For Roger, it was reassuring for his family to know that he was "true to himself" despite being so sick.

When I ask people what's important to them at the end of their life, they will often tell me. The problem is, most people are never asked that question. When asked, they are remarkably specific. Some people say that they want to go to the ocean again, or go fishing one more time. For Roger, it was important to still go out to lunch and to tag sales with Lorraine. Many people say that they want to be comfortable, free of symptoms, and remain in their own home. Once we know what's important to someone, families and hospice can often help to make those things happen. It can provide families with everlasting contentment.

Managing symptoms at the end of life usually involves both medication and non-medication approaches. There are several environmental measures that can help relieve difficulty breathing, such as having fresh or cooled air, using a circulating fan, sitting upright or even slightly forward, and wearing loose, unrestrictive clothing. Social and emotional measures can also help. For example, breathing exercises, pacing activities, distraction, relaxation, and calming music may be offered.[5]

Morphine helped Roger be comfortable and breathe better long before he died. It also helped him live more normally and enjoy going out with his wife. Morphine doesn't "kill" people, diseases do. If people wait until they are close to death to take an opioid medication, like morphine, sometimes it appears as if the morphine caused the death. It might just be that someone was finally comfortable enough to die. Morphine is a very important medication, not just for pain but also for shortness of breath.[6] Once all the usual medicines are used to help people breathe (steroids, water pills, cough medicines, oxygen, inhalers, etc.), the humane thing to do at the end of life is to give people morphine to prevent suffering and gasping for air. Many family members, and even health care staff, are afraid to administer morphine.[7] It's understandable given the significant problem of opioid addiction and overdose in our society. However, with end-stage diseases and associated symptoms that often occur, morphine relieves suffering and allows someone to die peacefully.[8]

CHAPTER 10

# Managing Anxiety and Restlessness

All her life, Sandy has known that she marches to a different tune, is on a different wavelength, and sees the world from a different perspective. She is an artist who uses materials from nature to create intricate wall hangings and sculptures. Sandy grew up the third of four daughters in an old farmhouse where she and her wife, Amy, now live. The house resembles a house from a children's storybook. Vines crawl up the red clapboard side of the house toward the roof. Large vertical windows line the face of the house, and wide cement stairs, covered with potted plants, lead to an ornate, black wooden door. The door holds one of Sandy's whimsical sculptures, a circle of driftwood with spiny offshoots and dried mushrooms and feathers woven around the wooden wreath. The large yard, with sweeping oak and pine trees, and the acres of forest in the back, are both Sandy's refuge and source of creativity.

Inside the home is a large, open, and sunny great room full of plants, sculptures, mobiles, and art hangings. The high ceiling has large wooden beams and two skylights that cast white rectangles on each side of the room. Sandy sits on a large memory foam mattress up against the window, in the far corner of the room. Her view overlooks the side yard with apple and beech trees, several birdfeeders, and a rambling stone wall.

Sandy has surrounded her "nest" with everything she needs during the day: ice water in a large tumbler with a straw, a smoothie (made and packed in ice by Amy), tissues, various snacks, books, journals, her phone, her medicine, the commode, and plenty of pillows and fleece blankets. Her dog, Piper, a spaniel mix, and two sister cats, Lily and Lace, take their usual positions around the bed and window.

Two years ago, at the age of fifty-eight, Sandy was diagnosed with breast cancer. She was treated with surgery, chemotherapy, and radiation, but the cancer spread to her lungs. Thankfully, she doesn't have a lot of coughing or breathing problems, nor does she have much nausea or vomiting. Fatigue has really been the worst of it. Sandy manages that by resting, meditating, and doing energy work. A month ago, her doctor told her that the treatment doesn't seem to be working anymore and she now has a "spot" on her liver and right hip. They offered her more treatment, but the chances of it getting better were very low. She and her doctor discussed the benefits of radiation if the bone pain gets bad; otherwise, hospice, at this point, would benefit her the most. It has been a rough road, but she's grateful that she made it through another summer, her favorite season. "I love the buzz in the air, the flowers, and the warm sun," she told him. "I suppose I can be thankful for that."

Hospice has been coming to visit Sandy for the past two weeks. Her primary goal is to be as independent as possible and to finish a sculpture she is making for her niece. Sandy is managing things physically; she says the pain in her right hip is controlled with a pill, ice, and cannabis cream. The neighbor stops in after school and checks on her and lets Piper out. Amy calls mid-morning and afternoon. She spends her days mostly reading, dozing, and listening to prayer circles and other spiritual offerings on her phone.

Lately, Sandy's emotions run the gamut from acceptance to panic and desperation. She starts thinking about actually dying and her breathing becomes rapid; she feels a fluttering in her chest and her hands get clammy. She's been working on managing these episodes with paced breathing and a guided imagery app on her phone. She is adamant about not taking too much anti-anxiety medication because it makes her too drowsy. "It zaps all my energy and creativity," she says.

Sandy also refuses to have people with her throughout the day. Amy worries about her being by herself, but she also knows her all too well and supports her decision. "She knows she can call me or my sister anytime if she needs to."

Her nurse, Charlene, visits twice a week. She checks to see how Sandy is doing, helps her manage symptoms, reorders medications and supplies, and provides her with a lot of emotional support. Charlene is a certified reiki and energy work practitioner. Her visits include a discussion on ways to manage pain, worry, and anxiety. Charlene regularly offers visits by the hospice social worker and spiritual counselor, but up until now, Sandy has declined. She does have a hospice volunteer, Jill, who visits weekly. Jill is in her mid-sixties, with short, cropped white hair and soft hazel eyes. Each visit, she brings Sandy the weekly bulletin from church that Sunday. She reads Sandy the prayers, psalms, and short, inspiring quotes. Jill's calm disposition and peaceful presence help Sandy relax. Jill and her husband are avid birdwatchers, so she also shares beautiful pictures and stories of bird sightings with Sandy. Jill has been gently encouraging Sandy to work on the sculpture for her niece, offering to gather materials from the yard if needed. Sandy insists, "I have what I need already—I just have to free my mind enough to pull it together."

One morning, Charlene arrives at Sandy's house for a routine check-in. While she is gathering her supplies from her trunk, she hears Piper barking at the door. She knocks on the door, opens it, calls Sandy, and lets Piper out. Sandy is lying on her bed on her left side facing the window in the far corner of the room. Her right hand is spread out and grabbing her right hip and her left hand is covering her eyes. "Sandy, are you all right?" Charlene asks, moving quickly toward her bed. Sandy says nothing, just shakes her head.

Sandy's hair is light brown and has come in like peach fuzz since she stopped chemotherapy. The shorter hair makes her big brown eyes seem larger and more striking. Sandy has been crying. Her eyes and nose are wet and her cheeks are red. "My goodness, Sandy, what's going on?" Charlene asks as she reaches over and places her hand on Sandy's shoulder. "Is it your hip?"

Sandy wipes her eyes and dots her nose with a tissue. "My hip has been excruciatingly painful since last night; I hardly slept at all. I've been taking an oxycodone pain pill every four hours and it hasn't helped. I also tried the cannabis cream and an ice pack, but nothing is working."

Charlene immediately grabs the oxycodone medication bottle from the table near the bed and takes out a pill. "Here, Sandy," she says as she reaches over and passes her the cup with water. "Do you want to take one of your anti-anxiety pills? It will probably help you be calmer and might also relax your muscles some." Sandy readily accepts it this time.

After several minutes, Sandy repositions her pillows and stretches out her legs. "Feeling a little better?" Charlene asks. Sandy nods and closes her eyes. Charlene then asks Sandy a number of questions about her symptoms and medications so she can call the hospice doctor and strategize on a better pain management plan.

"Sandy, have you been taking the steroid, dexamethasone, that the doctor ordered for the bone pain and swelling?"

Sandy squints and taps her index finger on her lips as she recalls, "No, I haven't. That's the pill that makes me too jumpy; I couldn't sleep at all after I took that pill."

"That's okay," Charlene says. "Sometimes, though, you take medication for one effect and then have to add another medication to counteract the side effects of the first one." Charlene goes on to explain, "For example, dexamethasone is really helpful for bone pain, and adding a medication like lorazepam can help with relaxation and sleep.[1] Also, opioid pain pills are notoriously constipating. Taking bowel medicine can counteract the side effects of the pain pills."[2]

Sandy sits up a little in bed and blows her nose. "I don't want to take all these pills if I can avoid it. At least the oxycodone used to take the edge off, but I don't like the way the dexamethasone makes me feel."

"That's fine, Sandy," Charlene says as she reaches over and rubs her shoulder. "If you don't want to take the dexamethasone, you can take ibuprofen instead, so long as you take it with something to eat."

"I'd much rather do that," Sandy agrees.

"You know, Sandy, cancer tends to grow and interfere with movement and comfort. It's not uncommon to need higher doses of pain medicine over time.[3] It's better to get ahead of the pain by taking scheduled medicine around the clock, instead of waiting until the pain gets bad and then playing catchup. I think it would be a good idea for you to consider starting on a pain patch," Charlene offers tentatively.

"You put the patch on your upper arm or chest, and it works around the clock on the pain. You change it every three days. If you have any breakthrough pain, then you can take one of the oxycodone pills."[4]

"I guess I can try it, as long as it doesn't knock me out."

"Well, it might take a day or two to adjust to the new medicine, but it will definitely help you, both while you're awake and sleeping. Let's see what the doctor says."

Charlene calls the doctor and reports the increase in Sandy's hip pain. She agrees with the plan to start a fentanyl patch. She also orders an increase in Sandy's dose of the short-acting oxycodone pills, just in case she needs them. Charlene relays this new information to Sandy. She also suggests that Sandy take an ibuprofen pill now and put a new ice pack on her hip. As she heads to the kitchen to gather both, she notices Piper sitting on the front step waiting to come in. When she opens the door, Piper scurries over to Sandy, wagging her tail. "Come here, you little nugget," she hears Sandy calling to Piper. She jumps up on the bed, circles around, and nestles herself in the fleece blanket.

When Charlene returns, she places the ice pack under Sandy's right hip and fluffs up her pillow. She gently grabs Sandy's hand and leads her through a deep breathing exercise. Sandy follows Charlene's lead and closes her eyes and takes deep breaths. Charlene feels the shift in Sandy's relaxation as she watches her chest and belly rise and fall. "Breathe in through your nose, and out your mouth," she softly tells Sandy. "Smell a rose; blow out a candle." Charlene releases Sandy's hand and extends her arms and hands over Sandy's right hip, just above the skin. She holds them there, giving her a reiki treatment, as Sandy settles in and rests.

The next morning, Charlene calls Sandy to check in. "I'm doing okay, I guess. I definitely slept better last night," Sandy tells her. "Amy is home today and making me some breakfast right now."

Charlene reiterates the instructions regarding the plan for managing the pain. Once again, she lets Sandy know that following the plan should make the pain better, but if she doesn't want to take something, or if the plan isn't working, she should let Charlene know. "I would rather you call us and tell us what's going on rather than walking in again to find you in terrible pain."

"Okay, I will," Sandy promises.

Over the next month, Sandy is "holding her own." Charlene and Jill visit regularly, providing care, guidance, and support. Sandy and Jill have been working on the sculpture for Sandy's niece. Sandy found the most interesting piece of driftwood when she and Amy were last at the beach. The whole piece is about a foot long and six inches tall. The left side has four spiny branches that intertwine and shoot up and to the right. It almost has the look of a bonsai tree without the leaves. The right side of the base has a shallow bowl in the wood. Sandy has taken several small, smooth glass stones that are clear, light blue, and dark blue, and has glued them into the bowl. She still has to carve the wood a bit more in the back and then hang something from the branches to make it look more like a shaded tree. "I feel better being able to work," she tells Jill. "I feel useful for a change." Sandy also now feels hopeful that the piece will be finished before her niece's birthday in October.

During one of Charlene's usual visits, Sandy relays an episode of anxiety, "even panic," that happened over the weekend.

"That sounds terrible, Sandy."

"It was. Amy was out at the grocery store. I started thinking about dying and about this house, how long it's been in the family, and the sadness that my illness has brought to this home." As Sandy talks, her eyes circle around the large great room and then settle back on her hands. "It was awful. I was claustrophobic and couldn't breathe. I called Amy and she came right home."

"I'm so sorry, Sandy."

"Amy and I had a long talk, Charlene. I don't want to die here. I love this house and this yard, but I have too many memories, too much sadness. It's like everything is rushing past me and I can't figure anything out."

"This is a lot, Sandy."

"I know Amy would take leave from work and care for me with help from my sisters, but I think it would be better if I had medical people around who are used to all this. I just don't feel like we can handle this. At least I can't."

"That's fine, Sandy."

"You mentioned about that hospice house. I think it would be better if I go there."

Sandy and Charlene talk about what that would be like, when she would want it to happen, and how arrangements are made. Charlene reassures Sandy that she supports her decision, whatever it is.

"I want to go, but I don't," Sandy says as tears well up in her eyes. "I've been thinking and worrying about this for a while and, to be honest, I'm actually relieved that I've decided."

Charlene and Sandy talk more about the details, the tradeoffs, and the emotions involved with this decision. "Amy will be able to stay over with you, Sandy. They even let your pets visit," Charlene reassures her. She lets Sandy know that it's the social worker with hospice who usually helps make arrangements when people move to a new location. She will ask their social worker, Pat, to call and arrange a meeting with both Sandy and Amy.

Over the next two weeks, Amy visits Cicely's Home Hospice and takes pictures for Sandy to see where she'll be moving. "Everyone is incredibly nice, Sandy. All the rooms are large with a big window overlooking the yard."

Charlene and Pat make a visit together one last time to arrange the details for Sandy's transfer to the residential hospice. They reassure Sandy and Amy that the hospice team there will take good care of them. "We work with them a lot," Pat tells them. "You will be in good hands."

"Oh," Sandy says to Amy as Charlene and Pat are getting ready to leave, "show them the finished product!" Amy leaves the room, and when she returns, she's carefully carrying a wooden structure. Sandy proudly shows them the sculpture that she finished with Jill's help. "We added miniature hemlock pine cones to the knotty areas and the ends of the spiny branches. I even added a small bird in the tree for Jill, made out of tiny feathers," she smiles. From a distance, it looks like a shaded tree overlooking a glistening pond. It looks incredibly peaceful, they all agree.

## REFLECTIONS ON SANDY AND FAMILY

Sometimes it seems that people like Sandy, who are artistic and creative, feel things on many levels. It can be overwhelming. One of the most surprising lessons I learned when I first started doing hospice work is how common anxiety and restlessness are. There is a lot of change and uncertainty. Sometimes the causes are physical, such as pain or difficulty breathing. Other times, it's related to worry, fear, and the unknown. One of the most difficult parts of being sick and dying is "the unknown." Going through treatment and not knowing whether it's working, or if the disease is getting worse despite treatment, can be nerve-wracking. Slowly approaching death and not knowing what to expect or where you're actually going when you die can be deeply troublesome. This was particularly hard for Sandy. It's normal to have a range of emotions during this sad and stressful time. Thankfully, there are many interventions that can help with anxiety and restlessness. Medicines can de-escalate severe symptoms. Therapies such as music, energy work, touch, and guided imagery can also help.[5] Talking with a social worker, spiritual counselor, or a loved one can help clarify beliefs and values that might provide a firmer sense of the path forward and beyond.[6]

Everyone is different. What each person wants when they're dying and how they want to spend their time varies. Some people want a lot of people around when they're sick and other people, like Sandy, like to be alone. When lots of family and friends do visit, it's important to give the person time to rest. If someone prefers more time alone, it can be a challenge for families to determine how much help to give someone so they can still stay safe and well cared for. Some people at the end of their life are content to stay home with loved ones for the time they have left. Other people feel better about themselves when they're doing something familiar and productive. It makes them feel like they're who they really are, despite their illness. For Sandy, she felt better when she was being creative.

## CHAPTER 11

# I Just Can't Do This Anymore

Charlene pulls into the driveway of the home Judith shares with her daughter Lisa. The small gray house has faded white trim, broken shingles, and a rusty drainpipe that leads into a cracked white plastic pail. Charlene grabs her supplies from her trunk and heads toward the side entrance of the house. She knocks on the door that has a big red STOP sign on it that reads: "No Smoking, Oxygen in Use." Charlene knows that Judith can't get to the door by herself, so she enters and yells, "Hi, Judith. It's Charlene from hospice."

No answer, but that's not unusual. Judith's bedroom is at the back left side of the house off the hallway. Charlene walks through the kitchen where all the counters and the small table at the far end of the kitchen are stacked with food, papers, mail, containers, and a variety of other household items. As Charlene heads down the hallway toward the bathroom and bedrooms, she notices oxygen tubing on the floor running from Judith's bedroom on the far left, diagonally to the bathroom, the first door on the right.

"Judith?" Charlene calls to her so she doesn't startle her. When Charlene turns into the bathroom, she finds Judith sitting on the toilet, leaning left as far as she can to keep the oxygen tubing in her nose. She is in terrible distress, panting in order to breathe. "Oh, my goodness, Judith, let me help you," Charlene says as she quickly grabs the wheelchair and helps Judith back to her bedroom. There she switches the oxygen over to a face mask, turns on the fan, and sets up a nebulizer treatment. Charlene checks the plastic pill boxes to see if Judith has taken the medicine that her daughter sets up for her. This morning's container is empty.

Judith is sitting in the wheelchair up against her bed holding on to the oxygen face mask with one hand and clutching a tissue in her lap with the other. She is seventy-four years old and doesn't weigh much more than seventy-four pounds. Her straight black and gray hair looks thin and wet behind the mask and the elastic strap that wraps around her head. In contrast, Judith's skin is white and paper thin, with several red bruises and superficial skin tears on her forearms and on the front of her legs. She is still breathing with her entire upper body moving forward in the wheelchair, but her breathing rate is slowing down. "Are you doing a bit better?" Charlene asks as she bends over to meet Judith's eyes. She nods. After checking her vital signs, Charlene sets up the breathing treatment and hands her the mouthpiece. "Here you go, Judith. I'm going to take a minute and call Lisa at work."

This is exactly the scenario that the hospice team feared. Judith's daughter Lisa works forty-five minutes away and has been adamant that her mother not receive any morphine or lorazepam. Judith has been living with Lisa for the past nine months. Their relationship is complicated and emotional. Judith was a single parent who raised her three children by working a variety of jobs, mostly waitressing. She has a long history of smoking cigarettes and drinking alcohol excessively. Her drinking and absenteeism caused her to lose several jobs over the years. She was in detox and rehab a couple of times, but eventually she would go back to the same haunts, and the same crowd, and inevitably start drinking again.

When her son, David, was a senior in high school, he was killed in a one-car accident in the early morning hours. It was determined that alcohol and speed were involved in the crash. Judith was crushed. According to Lisa, from that point on, she "packed it in." She was drinking heavily and started abusing sedatives. Lisa and her sister, Joanne, and Judith's sister, Chris, got her into a program for women that focuses on people in crisis who are dually diagnosed, both with mental illness and substance use disorder. The program seemed like it was a perfect fit; it focused on medication-assisted therapy, counseling, and integrative therapies. Judith went through the program but was always edgy and restless and appeared disinterested. She was treated for depression and referred to an outpatient program for counseling and support. Not long after getting out of the inpatient program, Judith began drinking again and taking a number of drugs to numb her pain. It was then that her daughter, Joanne, broke off contact with her mom. They had had one too many fights over her drinking, drugs, and not taking care of herself. In the last few years, Judith has been hospitalized numerous times with COPD. After the last hospitalization with pneumonia, respiratory failure, and weight loss, Judith was referred to hospice care.

Charlene is waiting on hold to speak with Lisa at work. She looks at Judith and then reaches over and gently rubs her upper back. Judith's hands are shaking a little, but she is still holding the nebulizer mouthpiece. "Are you still getting the medicine?" Charlene asks. Judith nods.

"Hi, Lisa, I'm here with your mom; she's not doing very well," Charlene reports. "When I came over, she was in terrible distress and couldn't breathe. She's doing a bit better now, but she's still breathing heavily, about thirty-four breaths per minute, and her oxygen level is low, only eighty-six percent. She's really suffering and would benefit from a low dose of morphine." Charlene braces herself for Lisa's refusal. "I'm happy to stay with her for an hour or so afterward to make sure she is okay," Charlene offers.

"What did she do? Did she forget to take her medicine again? Are you sure she took her steroid this morning?" Lisa asks with a tone of annoyance.

"The medicine container for this morning is empty," Charlene reports. "Lisa, I've done all the usual emergency measures I can to help your mom breathe, but she needs more. I would like to give her a very small dose of morphine from the emergency kit to see if it helps, and I will stay with her until you get home."[1]

Although Judith has the capacity to make her own decisions, she is timid and defers to her daughter. Charlene prefers to get Lisa's okay, since she is Judith's primary caregiver and their relationship and circumstances are so complicated. Lisa agrees, perhaps because she senses that Charlene is adamant about relieving Judith's difficulty breathing, or she is in a hurry to get off the phone. Either way, she tells Charlene that she will be home as soon as she can.

Charlene goes into the refrigerator and opens up the emergency medicine kit where she finds prefilled doses of morphine. She grabs one of the oral syringes and heads back to Judith's room. Judith is breathing deeply with one hand holding her forehead and the other one holding the nebulizer hose and mouthpiece in her lap.

"It looks like the nebulizer medicine is all done; let me take this out of your way," Charlene says as she grabs the apparatus from Judith and wraps the hose and mouthpiece around the machine. "Judith, I'm going to give you a small dose of this morphine; it should help your breathing." Charlene takes the syringe and squirts half of the dose into her mouth. Judith quickly shuts her eyes tight and sticks out her tongue. "I know," Charlene says, "it doesn't taste that good, but it will help. Here, take a little sip of water."

After twenty minutes, Judith's breathing becomes noticeably easier and more relaxed. Her breathing rate comes down to twenty-six and she is now able to talk in short sentences. She asks for a small glass of diet orange soda, which Charlene gets for her. Charlene asks if she'd like to get into her bed for a while, but Judith declines, saying she'd rather sit up in her recliner instead. Judith's large maroon recliner sits diagonally in the opposite corner of her room. Charlene moves the wheelchair up kitty-corner to the recliner, watching carefully for the oxygen tubing, and then helps Judith transfer into her chair. *Oh dear, she is light as a feather; all I can feel are bones.* Charlene puts on the television for Judith, takes out her laptop, and begins to chart.

When Lisa gets home, she comes right into the back bedroom where her mom and Charlene are sitting. She quickly takes off her coat, throws it on the bed, and fires questions to her mother, "What did you do? Did you forget to take your inhaler? Ma, I can't be running back here all the time; I'll lose my job if I do." Judith tries to answer Lisa's questions by nodding and shaking her head yes and no while glancing back and forth between Lisa and Charlene.

Charlene reiterates how she found her and what she's had for treatments so far. "Thankfully, she's doing a lot better. Lisa, I think it might be time to talk about where your mother is at and what might be helpful for both of you at this point. Is there a time tomorrow when we can meet with our social worker, Pat, and talk about ways we might be able to help?" Charlene asks tentatively.

Lisa takes a deep breath, shakes her head back and forth, but agrees to meet the next day since she is off from work anyway. Relieved, Charlene confirms the time with both Lisa and Judith, then writes down instructions on what to do if her breathing gets bad again. She also pleads with them to please call hospice right away if Judith is in any distress.

The following day, Charlene and Pat arrive just as Judith is finishing lunch. Her diet is now just a small amount of soft foods: peaches, half a banana, and a small scoop of sherbet. She gets short of breath easily with just eating and talking. Judith is sitting up in her recliner with her oxygen on and the portable table over her lap. Her breathing is a bit fast, but she tells them that she is not feeling short of breath. Pat introduces herself as the hospice social worker who is there to see what she can do to secure more care for Judith and to support them both with all the changes they are going through.

Pat reviews what services are available from hospice and from the elder service agency in the area. "I know it's really hard when someone gets sicker and needs more care; it's hard on everyone," she acknowledges.

As they all talk about options, Lisa's responses are blunt and decisive: "We aren't having tons of people coming and going. We can't afford to have someone here all the time." Pat tries to engage Judith in the discussion, but she just nods slightly; her eyes look like a frightened kitten. All of a sudden, she begins to cough, covering her mouth with a tissue as her eyes open wide and tear up.

Charlene rolls the portable table away from Judith and hands her a pillow to hug while she coughs. Pat and Lisa both stand up, ready to help in some way. After a few seconds, Judith begins to recover from the coughing jag but her mouth is open and she is breathing deeply. She dabs her eyes with a tissue. Charlene directs Lisa to grab the bottle of cough medicine on the dresser. She then pours the syrup into the medicine cup and passes it to Judith. Charlene reaches over and steadies Judith's hand as she helps guide the cup to her mouth.

Looking at Judith, then at Lisa, Charlene says, "I think it would be best if your mom takes the second half of the morphine dose from yesterday. This will help her breathing a lot."

"That's fine." Lisa says as she sits on the edge of the bed. She takes a deep breath, exhales deeply, and then lets her head fall back onto the bed. "I just can't do this anymore."

"Well, we're going to help you, Lisa," Pat reassures her. She explains that hospice offers a respite benefit, whereby people can be transferred to a facility, usually a nursing home, for up to five nights. This allows families to regroup and discuss ongoing plans for care. Some families set up additional care at home, and sometimes people stay at the facility beyond the five days. "It will give you time to sort out what's needed, and then we'll help you figure out what's best for you both."

Lisa acknowledges that these last few episodes were scary. "I'm glad you were here," she says. Charlene looks at Lisa and realizes how tired and worried she looks. These past nine months have taken a toll on her and it shows. Judith is now sitting back in the recliner with her eyes closed and her head resting on the headrest. She looks so much more comfortable.

After further discussion and several phone calls, Lisa and Judith opt for a respite stay for Judith at Woodland Hills Nursing Home. The ambulance comes and takes Judith there. Soon afterward, Charlene arrives and confers with the nursing home staff on Judith's medications and the plan of care. She also arranges for a hospice volunteer and home health aide to visit with Judith at the nursing home, to give her some one-on-one care and attention.

The aide, Luz, gives Judith a good sponge bath and helps keep her tender skin clean and moist. The volunteer, Maria, sits quietly with her and keeps her company. Maria realizes that she and Judith have both worked for the same restaurant, only at different times. She takes the time to learn just who Judith is beneath all the pain and sadness. She discovers that Judith used to write poetry when she was a teenager and in her early twenties. She even won a poetry contest sponsored by the local library. Judith also tells Maria that she loves animals, but she hasn't been able to have a pet since her children were little. She acknowledges that she had a hard enough time taking care of herself, never mind an animal. Each visit, Maria reads poetry to Judith from collections by Mary Oliver and John O'Donohue. One Sunday afternoon, Maria surprises Judith by bringing her black Lab, Molly, to visit. Judith smiles as she nuzzles her face against Molly's big head and scratches her back.

Over these five days, it becomes clear to Lisa that she can't provide the around-the-clock care that her mother now needs. She is relieved to learn that her mother is eligible for nursing home coverage and that hospice will continue to visit her at Woodland Hills. Now when she visits her mother, she can just be the daughter and not have to worry about how to manage emergencies. Judith is also adjusting pretty well to living at the nursing home. She tells Charlene that she feels good knowing that the nurses are there all the time in case she can't breathe.

Carole, the hospice spiritual and bereavement counselor, is also visiting her regularly to help her sort out all the sorrow and regrets that have weighed heavily on her heart and soul. They have deep conversations about suffering and pain, and how to achieve peace in this life before death.

Pat reaches out to Judith's estranged daughter, Joanne, to update her on her mother's situation and to see if she wants to visit with her mother at the nursing home. Pat offers to be there with them if it would help provide some structure and boundaries. Joanne says that she would like to visit and reconcile with her mother, and perhaps at another visit bring her two kids in to see her. "It might help us all heal," she tells Pat.

When Pat goes back into Judith's room to let her know about the upcoming visit with Joanne, Maria is reading a Mary Oliver poem to Judith, who is resting back in her recliner with her eyes closed: "Truly we live with mysteries too marvelous to be understood."[2]

## REFLECTIONS ON JUDITH AND FAMILY

Many families deal with substance use, violence, trauma, and loss. Relationships between family members can be tense, explosive, or estranged. Hospice doesn't take sides and demonize anyone, nor do they try to solve long-standing family difficulties; rather, they try to hold up families as they go through the loss of a loved one. Sometimes families have an opportunity to express regret, sorrow, and forgiveness, and sometimes they don't. I've found that most families, regardless of their relationship difficulties, want their loved one to be comfortable and have a peaceful death. It's not unusual, however, to have mixed and complicated feelings after someone dies when there was a long history of family discord. The experience of grief often involves reflecting on the relationship, experiences, and feelings involved with the person who died.[3]

Many people get sick because of things they do or because of the way they live, such as smoking cigarettes or eating foods that aren't good for them. The end of life is not the time to blame people for unhealthy behavior. There are many factors that cause people to live the way they do. Underneath medical, social, and personal problems is often an individual who has suffered trauma and loss and has tried to deal with it in a number of ways, both healthy and unhealthy.

Most people say that they want to die at home. Sometimes this happens and many times it doesn't.[4] It was hard to know what Judith and Lisa really wanted. Sometimes family members feel an obligation to "take in" loved ones when they are sick. Other times, people don't realize how much work and how emotional it can be to care for someone who is dying. Hiring 24/7 help is difficult and unaffordable for most families. Hospice residences and nursing homes charge for room and board, and some people don't have insurance coverage for that. These decisions can be heart-wrenching for families. The hospice benefit includes a number of short-term emergency and respite services. Hospice can help families access these services. Also, hospice team members can support families as they deal with these difficult decisions and emotions.

CHAPTER 12

# Nothing Left Unsaid

Linda is sitting in her living room basking in the sun and warmth of her condo on a Saturday afternoon. She carefully puts her handmade bookmark, crafted by one of her former students, into her book, takes off her glasses, and rubs her eyes while taking a deep sigh. Two years ago, Linda retired from teaching middle school English and moved into this retirement community. She glances around the apartment scanning her prized possessions: photographs of her two children over the years, a collection of awards and photos, especially her etched-glass "Teacher of the Year Award," and her large collection of favorite books. Linda's eyes focus on a photograph of her with her sister, Betty, at the beach when they were about eight and ten years old, respectively. *I loved that little yellow bathing suit with the skirt*, she thinks as her mind drifts away to her youth and memories of summers gone by. *How am I going to tell Betty and the kids about what's going on? I'm not even sure I know what's going on.* After a few minutes, Linda snaps to, focuses sharply on the hands of the kitchen clock that say 3:10 p.m., and realizes that she better get up and get ready for church before her older sister Betty arrives.

Betty is a retired nurse and now lives in the next town over. Since they have both retired, Linda and Betty started a ritual of going to church together on Saturday afternoons, then having dinner together, alternating at each other's home. This is Linda's week to host dinner and the pot roast and vegetables are in the slow cooker ready to go.

After returning from church, Linda and Betty bustle around the kitchen setting the table, preparing supper, and carrying on the usual conversation about the sermon, whom they saw in church and what they wore, and who wasn't there. They fill their plates, share compliments on the meal, shake their napkins and cover their laps, and slowly settle into the silence as Betty says grace. Linda takes one bite of her potato and abruptly puts down her fork. She rushes into the bathroom and vomits. Later on, once her stomach has settled, she begins to tell Betty what's been going on. Two weeks ago, she started to feel a strange, dull pain in her stomach, "like a knot." Since then, she has lost her appetite and has even felt nauseated off and on. "I think something serious might be going on. How am I going to tell Tina and Tim?" Linda worries as she looks down at her hands that are neatly smoothing and folding a tissue in her lap.

Betty listens carefully and offers her encouragement, just like she always has. "Let's just take it one day at a time, starting with calling your doctor on Monday."

Linda calls her doctor's office and thankfully gets an appointment for the next day. She decides to go to this appointment by herself. *Why worry anybody else at this point? It could be nothing.* At the doctor's appointment, Linda tries to gauge how worried she should be based on the doctor's questions and comments. She's only been seeing this doctor for two years. He is serious and businesslike but thorough. Linda misses her longtime doctor who retired two years ago, especially now. This new doctor asks a lot of questions about her diet and her nausea and vomiting episodes. He looks carefully at Linda's eyes and in her mouth. He also presses gently on her belly for what seems like a long time. Linda can feel her heart quicken as she waits in anticipation of what he concludes from all this.

"I'm going to order some bloodwork and an ultrasound of your liver, just to rule out anything serious. I'm also sending over a prescription to your pharmacy for an anti-nausea medication. That should help."

"Okay," Linda says, too stunned and worried to ask any more questions. Her mind is racing.

*What could be wrong with my liver? What does your liver do anyway? I wonder why he was looking in my eyes and in my mouth, then. I better tell Tina and Betty; they would want to know. Oh dear, and what about Tim?*

Linda talks on the phone with her daughter, Tina, at least every other day, and they see each other at least every week or two. Tina works in the admissions department at a local community college. Linda is thrilled to have Tina live nearby again. After college, Tina moved down south where she met her husband, Dan. They lived in North Carolina for years, but their marriage didn't work out, so three years ago, Tina moved back home.

They're closer than they've ever been. Tina helped Linda move into her apartment after she retired. It made downsizing so much easier. They go to a lot of events together. The college where Tina works has several concerts and guest lecturers; Linda is often invited as Tina's guest. Linda now enjoys the time she spends with her daughter. It is free from the strife of earlier times when Tina was in her teens and early twenties.

*Those days were tough. Two people fighting to hold on to who knows what.*

Linda's son Tim is a source of deep pain and sadness for Linda. Tim has an addiction to painkillers and has been in and out of jail two or three times. Linda has tried to help him in so many ways. She worries about him all the time.

Linda tells Tina and Betty about the doctor's appointment and what tests have been ordered. They ask more questions than Linda has answers for. They both insist on going with her to whatever appointments she has. She's relieved. This is all very frightening.

"Tina, I know you don't get along with Tim, but I need to call him," Linda says tentatively.

"Why? He only calls you when he needs money. I don't know why you keep bailing him out. You're not doing him any favors, you know."

Tina is fed up with her brother. She hates the way he treats her mother and is tired of his endless crises. Every time Linda and Tina talk about Tim, the conversation ends in the same argument. Linda ends up feeling heartsick and withdraws. She lies down on her bed, grabs her rosaries from her headboard, and weeps silently.

The following day, Linda tries to call Tim at the number he last called from; there's no answer and no voicemail. She finds a number she has for a counselor he saw recently. She leaves a message for him to call. That familiar worry about Tim now takes on added weight.

Over the course of the next two weeks, Linda has numerous blood tests, doctor's appointments, scans, biopsies, and medications. These all confirm her worst fears. At the age of sixty-five, Linda is diagnosed with liver cancer and given a life expectancy of two to three months.

The next month is a whirlwind. Her emotions range from anger at being cheated out of years of retirement, to fear of dying and death, to profound sadness at losing time with Tina and Tim. She is also exhausted. Linda goes from seeing her regular doctor, to a liver doctor, to a cancer doctor. Everyone is ordering blood tests and other tests, poking her abdomen, shining lights into her eyes, asking her the same questions over and over. She sits in waiting rooms with loud and annoying daytime shows blaring on the television in the corner of the room. *Why am I doing all this? Is this going to make me live longer? Is this going to make me feel better?* Right then and there, she tells Tina that she isn't going to fight this anymore. "Nothing is helping anyway. All this is just making me tired and sick. I just want to go home to my sunny apartment."

Linda's disease progresses rapidly. She becomes weak and jaundiced. Tina takes a medical leave of absence and moves in to care for her mom. Betty comes over to help every afternoon. Tim's former counselor calls back and leaves a number for them to try to reach Tim.

It has only been a month since her last series of tests, when Linda decided to stop all treatments and call in hospice. The hospice team helps her with her medications, gives her a sponge bath, runs errands for Tina, and talks with them about what to expect in the weeks and days ahead, and about the emotional and spiritual worries they face.

Now Linda lies in a hospital bed in her sunny living room. The nurse, Charlene, sits at Linda's bedside with Tina and Betty. She explains to them why Linda's skin is such a dark gold color and why her belly and legs are so swollen. She shows them what to do with the urine bag and how to empty it. Charlene describes Linda's state of mind and how they should interact with her. "Hospice refers to this as 'unresponsive,' " she explains. "Even though she isn't able to talk and isn't awake, you should keep talking with her because she might still be able to hear you and experience your presence."[1]

Tina and Betty tell her what they are about to do, such as when they moisten her lips and when they are about to turn her over in bed. They also tell her that they love her and they thank her for being a good mom and sister.

The following afternoon, Tina is in the bathroom when she hears moaning coming from the living room. She quickly goes in and notices that her mom is moving her arms up and down and turning her head side to side. "Mom, are you okay? What's going on?" Tina asks nervously. Betty comes in from the kitchen and joins her at Linda's bedside. They each reach for her hand and try to console her. Linda continues to be restless and "in another state." After conferring on what else to do, they decide to call hospice.

The hospice nurse on call takes the report, asks a number of questions, and then encourages Tina to give her mom some of the prefilled medication for pain and restlessness. Tina goes into the refrigerator and grabs the medication as instructed. Betty raises up the head of the bed slightly and holds Linda's head still while Tina squirts two liquid medicines under her tongue with an oral syringe. "Here you go, Mom. This should help you feel better," Tina tries to reassure her. Tina and Betty remain on either side of the bed. They try to comfort her while also wondering what else they should do.

After what feels like hours but is only thirty minutes, Linda is still moaning and moving her arms and head around. Betty encourages Tina to call hospice back. "She needs something else, hon; she can't go on like this." When Tina calls the hospice nurse back, she says she will be right over.

Tina tells Betty what the nurse said as she's sitting at her mom's bedside trying to calm her down. "Even though I'm a retired nurse, it's hard to know what to do," Betty says to Tina. "It's hard when it's your sister and she is in pain." Tina's eyes well up as she thinks about the collective pain and sadness she feels for herself, her mother, and her aunt, and at the same time, she feels her eyes burn from so little sleep in the past week.

When the on-call nurse, Marie, arrives, she is updated by Tina and Betty and then assures them that she will help Linda to be more comfortable. "First I'll check some of the physical signs." She scans Linda's forehead with a thermometer. "No fever." Marie then listens to her chest and reports, "Her heart rate is fast, which is not unusual. I don't hear a lot of congestion in her lungs, which is good." She checks to see if Linda has passed any urine in the bag so far today; there was a small amount. After everything checks out, Marie gives her some more of the medicine for pain and restlessness.

Within fifteen minutes, the additional medicine seems to take effect, and Linda's body relaxes some. Her head has stopped moving, and her arms are more limp by her side. Tina and Betty sigh with relief. The three women gently wash Linda, put skin cream on her back, and moisten her lips with mouth swabs dipped in cool water.

Marie tells them that emotional distress is common for people at the end of life.[2] "Do you think she is worried about anything? Could she be waiting for anyone or anything?"

Silence fills the room. Tina and Betty look at each other and then Tina begins. "Well, my brother has been somewhat estranged from the family. He hasn't talked with my mom in months."

"Do you think your mom might be waiting to say goodbye to him?"

"I'm not sure; she might be," Tina says. Betty remains quiet, but her eyes well up with tears.

"Do you know if he can be reached?" Marie asks, looking over at Tina and then at Betty.

Betty cautiously offers, "Last we knew, he was in California. He's had a lot of problems. It's been very difficult for my sister. I know she has a number where he might be able to be reached."

Betty offers to go into the kitchen and try to call Tim. From the living room, Tina and Marie can hear Betty's muffled voice. She walks quickly into the living room and places the phone up to Linda's ear. After a minute, Betty takes the phone back and whispers, "Thank you, Tim." She walks back toward the kitchen, talking softly, and then says goodbye.

Linda lies still and quiet. Her skin color nearly matches the light from the setting sun that now bathes her living room. They sit quietly at her bedside for several minutes. Finally Marie breaks the silence and asks, "I know she has been a devout Catholic; has she seen a priest yet?"

"Yes," Betty tells her. "Father Donnelly just came yesterday and gave her the Anointing of the Sick. It was so nice of him."

"Well, that's good. Perhaps the three of us can say a prayer together," Marie offers.

"She'd like that," Betty confirms. "Hail Mary was always Linda's favorite prayer." As they gather around Linda's bed, Betty and Tina reach down and gently hold her hands. They all begin to recite the Hail Mary, ". . . now, and at the hour of our death. Amen." At that very moment, Linda takes her last breath and dies.

## REFLECTIONS ON LINDA AND FAMILY

Linda's death at the end of this prayer was a profound and momentous experience. What allows someone to leave this world? For many of us who have been privileged to witness someone's death, it seems like being clean, comfortable, and peaceful helps. For some people who are dying, it seems important for them to hear their family members say goodbye, even if they're not fully awake. The relationship between loved ones can run very deep. Often spouses, and parents and their children, worry about each other during the dying process. Saying goodbye, and giving the dying person permission to die, can bring both everlasting peace.

"Closure" is often used to mean completing any unfinished business before you die.[3] People who are dying may worry about many things, such as finalizing their will or taking care of funeral arrangements. Sometimes it's important for them to be back home again. Many people die soon after arriving home from being in the hospital. Sometimes they need to see certain friends or relatives before they die. For some people, hearing "Thank you," "I'm sorry," or "I love you" seems to help. What I've found is that people often strive to be at peace—physically, socially, emotionally, and spiritually—before they die. Helping people take care of business and offering them reassurance, gratitude, love, and forgiveness can often provide them with peace.

There are many moments that bring families together in the final days of a loved one's life. These special times provide a peaceful setting and create fond memories. Music, prayers, and family rituals are examples of activities that bring people together and can provide a soothing and memorable experience for everyone.

CHAPTER 13

# Keeping Things Normal

"He won't wake up!" Jim frantically says on the phone to the hospice nurse, Charlene. "He's been asleep since seven o'clock last night!" Charlene calmly asks Jim if he's sure his father is breathing. "Yes, I'm sure he is," Jim answers quickly.

"Does he seem to be in any distress? Do you think he's in pain or having a hard time breathing?" Charlene asks.

"No, he's just lying there, but it's eleven a.m. and he hasn't gotten up since he went to bed last night," Jim says. "This is not like him at all."

Charlene tells Jim that sometimes this happens; it sounds worrisome, but what matters is that he seems comfortable right now. "He may need to catch up a bit on sleep," she tells him. "But why don't I come over and check him out and make sure he is okay." Jim readily accepts the offer for a visit.

Ed has been on hospice care for the past month. During his last hospitalization, his doctor told him that his kidney disease was getting significantly worse and that without dialysis, it would advance much more rapidly. Ed also has a long list of other medical problems including heart disease, atrial fibrillation, high blood pressure, high cholesterol, and arthritis. Despite all that, he has been managing pretty well.

Ed's wife died three years ago in the hospital from heart failure and pneumonia. Ed's two sons, Jim and Rick, are surprised that their dad is doing so well after their mom died. Then again, Ed acquired the nickname "Steady Eddie" because his coworkers at the manufacturing plant found that Ed never seemed to get ruffled when problems came up. His famous saying is "Let's just take it one day at a time."

Charlene arrives at Ed's white two-story colonial home on the main street in town. She picks up the local newspaper from the front porch and knocks on the door. She hears Ed's dog, Buddy, barking wildly, and Jim opens the door right away. Charlene greets Jim, passes him the newspaper, bends down to greet Buddy, and then enters the living room on the right. The room is dark from walnut wood trim and similarly colored hardwood floors. The shades on the three windows are pulled down halfway, allowing only a shadow of light in the room. Ed's leather recliner is empty in the far corner of the room. Buddy jumps up and settles into the chair.

"Is he still sleeping?" Charlene asks Jim.

"Yes, he hasn't moved a bit," Jim says. "He hasn't had any breakfast, or anything at all to eat either."

"Okay, well let's go up and check on him," Charlene says as she gathers up her nurses' bag and slings the strap over her shoulder. Jim leads Charlene up the sturdy wooden stairs and down the hallway to Ed's bedroom on the right. His room is small and dark. There are two windows with the shades pulled, two twin beds, a tall dresser, a bedside table, and a walker up against the bed. Ed is lying in the first bed with the blankets covering him up to his shoulders. "He looks like he is just sleeping," Charlene whispers to Jim. She watches him for a while without speaking as Jim looks back and forth between his dad and Charlene. Still whispering, she tells Jim, "I'm not sure if he is just 'making up for lost sleep time' or if this is a new stage for him. He's probably exhausted and needs his sleep, Jim. I'm happy, though, to wake him up and check his vital signs, just to make sure he is okay," Charlene offers.

Jim readily accepts. "If you don't mind, since you're here . . . I'd feel better knowing if he's okay."

Charlene gently reaches out her hand and puts it on Ed's shoulder. "Ed," she says softly. "Ed," she repeats, shaking his shoulder a bit. Ed slowly opens his eyes, blinking several times. He raises his head, looks at Charlene and then over her shoulder at Jim. "You were in a pretty deep sleep, Ed; we were a bit worried about you," Charlene tells him.

"Dad, are you okay?" Jim asks. Without saying anything, Ed nods slightly, still coming out of the fog of sleep.

"Ed, would it be okay if I check your vital signs?"

He looks up at Charlene and nods.

"Do you want a sip of water or do you need to pee first?"

He declines both, so Charlene proceeds to check his temperature, pulse, oxygen level, and blood pressure. "Everything seems to check out, Ed," Charlene says as she stoops down to talk with him. Are you having any pain or discomfort?"

This time, Ed answers "no" as he shakes his head and looks up at Jim.

"Dad, are you hungry? Do you want something to eat?"

"I could eat a little something," Ed says, still getting his bearings.

Jim takes a deep breath and exhales sharply. He smiles at Charlene, relieved. They both help Ed sit up, get to the toilet, and get dressed. With one person in front of him and one person behind him, Ed climbs down the stairs for the last time.

When Ed was first admitted to hospice, Charlene and Pat, the social worker, asked Ed what was most important to him. Without hesitating, he said, "Just to live my life as normally as I can." He said he wants to spend his days, as much as possible, the way he had been. Jim and Rick heard him loud and clear and have tried to honor his wishes. They don't want a lot of people coming and going, so they declined other hospice staff visits, except the nurse's.

Jim, the oldest, took a leave of absence from his engineering job in order to take care of his dad. It's strange how things work out. Jim got divorced a year and a half ago and moved back home. It was only supposed to be temporary, until he got a place of his own, but weeks became months, and now, he's still there. In retrospect, it's been a godsend. He's been able to take care of the house and yard, and when his dad got sick, he did errands and took him to medical appointments. These past several years have made Jim realize how much he's like his dad. He's gone through a lot of change: his mom dying, his daughter going away to school, the divorce, and now his dad being sick. He manages to take things one day at a time and also and doesn't get too ruffled. He's concluded that he and his dad are both handy, logical, and calm. It has made this time with him easy.

His younger brother, Rick, is very different. He's energetic, talkative, and impulsive at times. They've always gotten along okay, probably because they're four years apart. Rick comes over several times a week to give Jim a break, and he stays overnight when he doesn't have to work the next day. Rick's a firefighter in town who works twelve-hour shifts, three to four times a week. He keeps his dad up to date on all the emergency department news and town business. Ed was a longtime Lions Club member, so he and Rick know a lot of the same people. Rick and Ed are also big sports fans, so they are always watching a game on TV or catching up on teams and scores.

Jim and Rick keep up with Ed's routine as much as they can. They make him his usual breakfast, read him the morning paper, especially the obituaries and the sports page, watch his television shows with him, and, most importantly, help take care of his dog, Buddy. After Ed's wife died, Buddy, a terrier mix, became his constant companion. Whenever Ed sits in his recliner, without fail, Buddy jumps up on his lap.

Jim thinks back a lot to that initial hospice discussion. Even though they were talking about pretty sensitive topics, his father was very matter-of-fact and decisive about everything. Charlene was reviewing Ed's current medications and the medical procedures he was getting. She let him know that the hospice doctor will often make recommendations to stop some of the tests and medications, either because they won't have much benefit at this point in his disease or because they might cause him more harm than good.[1] Jim remembers his dad saying that he'd just as soon stop whatever wasn't needed. "I take enough pills as it is." Logical and practical, as usual.

One of the other topics that hospice brought up was whether they had decided on what they wanted for final arrangements. The social worker started it off by acknowledging that it's often a sensitive question, but that they needed to discuss it early on. Pat gently asked them, "Is there a funeral home or crematorium that you and your family have decided to use?" Without hesitation, Ed told them that he already had prearrangements. He and his wife had taken care of that years ago; he had a plot already paid for next to his wife. Jim remembers looking at his dad, wondering what else he might reveal about his mom's death or how he was doing, especially now, with his illness and starting on hospice. Instead, he just commented on what a nice job the funeral home did with his wife. "It made it a lot easier."

After that morning's sleeping incident, Ed isn't quite the same. Although nothing urgent happened, it's the beginning of another stage in his decline. They set up a hospital bed in the dining room that adjoins the living room and still allows him to watch the television. Ed is starting to spend more and more time in bed sleeping.

Neither son has much experience with bedside care, so with their father's permission, they allow a home health aide to come in three times a week to bathe him, put cream on his skin, and change his diaper. The aide, Luz, and Charlene also teach them safe and comfortable ways to feed, turn, and clean him. One day when Jim and Rick are both there, Charlene demonstrates how to change the diaper. With each of them on opposite sides of the bed, she shows them how to turn him side to side, pull up the middle section from underneath him, and then fasten each tab on his hips. Up until now, Ed was using pull-ups and mostly taking care of them himself. Despite them joking about "having all thumbs," Jim and Rick do fine. They keep stepping up each time there's a new task to do or a new skill to learn. They also keep up his routine. They read him the newspaper, put on his favorite television shows, and help Buddy up onto the bed.

Over the next two weeks, Ed goes from eating soups and toast to not taking anything solid at all. He opens his eyes but seems distant, and he isn't talking anymore. He never seems to have any pain. Luz is now coming every day to bathe, dress, and turn him. Charlene or another nurse visit every day to every other day.

Jim and Rick continue to talk to him; they reassure him that they will be okay, and that they will take care of everything, especially Buddy. They sit at his bedside and tell stories about playing little league and taking camping vacations to the lake; they joke about the funny incidents that became family legends. They trade stories, they laugh, and they tear up.

One morning Luz shows up as usual to care for Ed. Jim gives her a short report and then excuses himself to go up and take a shower. Luz fills the basin with warm water and begins to wash and shave Ed. She washes his chest, arms, legs, and privates, all the while talking to him and explaining what she's doing. Ed's skin looks pale and dry. His breathing is shallow, but he doesn't seem to be in any pain. She thinks to herself how thin he has become, especially over the last few weeks. Luz then puts special cream on his hips and bottom, and turns him to put on a clean diaper and pajamas. She positions Ed on his back, brushes the few hairs on his head to the side, and moistens his mouth with a sponge. Luz grabs the bed controls, raises the head of Ed's bed slightly, lowers the bed to the lowest position, and raises up the side rails. She then takes a deep breath, reaches her forearm up, wipes the sweat from her forehead, and then rolls up the soiled linen and carefully grabs the basin of soapy water.

As Luz is cleaning up the supplies in the bathroom and throwing the laundry in the washing machine, she hears Jim come into the kitchen. "His right hip is a little red, Jim; I put some cream on it and left the diaper unfastened on that side. It might be a good idea to keep him off that side for a while," Luz suggests.

"I will, Luz, thank you. I'll see you tomorrow."

When Luz walks back into the dining room, she looks at Ed and notices that he isn't breathing. He is lying still and quiet just as she left him minutes ago, except he's not breathing. "Jim, come in here, I think your dad has just died," she urgently calls over to him. They both stand on the same side of the bed. Jim's eyes are wide with fear and urgency. Luz gently reminds him, "It's okay."

Jim reaches for his dad's hand and Luz rests her hand on Ed's thigh. Buddy is curled up at the end of the bed. After several minutes, Jim breaks the silence, "Well, he's with my mom now."

## REFLECTIONS ON ED AND FAMILY

A lot of people who are dying, like Ed, just want life to be as normal as possible. Perhaps they don't want to be the center of attention, or they don't want all the focus to be on medical things. They might not want to face the dying process and all the emotions that go with it. It's not entirely possible for life to proceed as it was, but trying to keep some normalcy can provide comfort and familiarity.

It's not always easy for children to provide bedside care to their parents who are dying. It can be personal, embarrassing, or awkward. Some people learn how to do it and some people hire aides to do it. Jim and Rick learned how to do it. Perhaps they used to change their kids' diapers, or they're pragmatic, like their dad, and just do what's needed. Most people who die from an illness need bedside care. Also, protecting someone's privacy is important to maintaining their dignity.[2] Dining rooms and living rooms become bedrooms for people who are dying. Medical staff and delivery people visit often when someone is sick. Closing doors and shades, and keeping people clean and covered, are important measures for upholding someone's dignity.

Hospice engages people in many sensitive discussions, such as choices for burial and cremation services. They understand that these decisions are necessary but also delicate. These topics often involve family, culture, and religious beliefs, and are deeply personal. Ed and his family were incredibly practical. For some families, these conversations are very difficult. To actually have these overt conversations sometimes makes people realize that their loved one is really going to die. Many families are grateful that hospice opens up and guides this discussion. Sometimes, they learn what's already been arranged, or what their loved one wants. These discussions often take place over time and involve several people, but they are important decisions to make nonetheless.[3]

CHAPTER 14

# The Agony of Waiting for Dad to Die

One of George's earliest memories is sitting on his father's lap while he drove the tractor around the farm. Up there, he could see everything: the cows, the rows of corn, the chicken coop, and the barn. Now he finds himself flooded with memories of his parents, all the adventures with his siblings on the farm, 4-H Club, and showing cows at the fair. He also remembers all the emergencies, like when his brother cut his fingers on the rototiller, the time the coyotes got into the chicken coop, and, of course, the fire in the barn. As he sits in his chair on the front porch, George's mind wanders over these memories as if he needs to touch them all over again, in this new state of dying, in order to make sense of them all. Occasionally, he'll share a memory with Shirley, his wife of sixty-two years, but mostly it's his own private journey.

Overall, George feels a sense of achievement and satisfaction. He and Shirley and their kids have kept the farm going. When the milk business got too expensive to operate, George and his son, Chris, refocused the farm to selling Christmas trees and other plants and shrubs, as well as products from local growers, such as honey, fruit, and jams. It was a great decision at the time because George was diagnosed with Parkinson's disease right after that and his body just couldn't keep up with the demands of the cows and milk production.

It's hard to imagine, but that was already ten years ago. George is now eighty-seven years old and the Parkinson's disease has really advanced. He has also been diagnosed with high blood pressure, arthritis, and dementia. Five years ago, he had a hip replacement, and a year after that a pacemaker was inserted in his heart. Whenever anyone asks George how he's doing, he always responds, "I can't complain; no one would listen to me anyway."

Shirley is only two years younger than George, but she is mostly healthy and strong as an ox. After the children started school, she worked for years managing accounts for the water department in town. She also has helped on the business side with the farm. She too had a hip replacement two years ago but is moving around like nothing ever happened.

Shirley is in their large kitchen making lunch for herself and George. She loves this kitchen. Many years ago, they had the wall between the kitchen and the den taken down to make room for a long wooden table, benches, and a center island. The glass-paned cabinets give the room a nice country charm. Shirley insisted that parts of the old kitchen be retained, so the old brick fireplace was made into a bookcase. Shirley neatly slides the grilled, chopped ham sandwich from the frying pan onto the plate, cuts it in quarters, and pours a glass of milk for both of them.

When Shirley arrives on the porch carrying the lunches on a tray, she notices that George has fallen asleep; his head is tipped back and to the right. "George, sweetheart," she says to him as she takes the plate and glass off the tray and places them on the folding end table. George easily wakes up and sits upright as Shirley takes the towel off her shoulder and tucks it under George's chin. She pulls up a chair right next to George and carefully picks up his milk glass and holds it to his lips. George takes a few sips and then holds up his right hand as it shakes side to side. She passes George a triangle of the ham sandwich. With his hand shaking, he moves it to his mouth and takes a small bite from the tip. He chews and moves the small amount of sandwich around in his mouth for several minutes as his hand falls back into his lap holding the rest of the sandwich. "George, you're going to have to eat more than that if you want to keep up your strength," Shirley says firmly as she holds up another piece of sandwich to his mouth. George shakes his head but points to the milk, hoping to settle for some middle ground.

"I just don't have an appetite," George says, his voice hoarse. He has already lost a lot of weight. His blue work pants are falling off him and his belt has already moved two holes. Shirley and their daughter Kim keep pushing him to eat more and he just can't.

"I'm going to go in and lie down," George tells Shirley as he pulls the towel down onto his lap. Shirley takes a deep breath and exhales with her lips closed tight. She rolls up the towel from George's lap, takes a quick bite of the sandwich herself, and moves the folding table away from him.

Shirley grabs the walker that's adjacent to his chair and squares it with him and the chair.

Standing to George's side, Shirley bends down and grabs ahold of his belt, and says, "Ready?" Without saying anything, George grabs both arms of the chair and pushes down with his hands and feet while Shirley helps him stand up. He stands, but his arms and knees are shaking and he's bent forward over the walker. "Stand up, George, and get your bearings," Shirley tells him. After several minutes, with

Shirley behind him still holding onto his belt, George shuffles, only an inch or two at a time with his walker, toward his bedroom.

Later that afternoon, while George is sleeping, Shirley is in the kitchen listening to the television while she peels and cuts up vegetables for dinner. She hears her daughter Kim come through the front porch door and sees her two grandchildren running out back in the yard. "Hi, Grammy!" they both yell as Shirley waves and smiles to them from the kitchen window.

Kim comes in and kisses her mom on the cheek while she is still at the sink peeling carrots. "Where's Dad?" she asks.

"He's taking a nap," Shirley tells her. "He's been awfully tired today."

"Well, how long has he been sleeping? Don't you think you should wake him up? He won't sleep tonight if he keeps on sleeping. Did he eat breakfast and lunch okay?"

Shirley grabs the dish towel hanging on the oven handle and dries her hands. She feels the weight of all these decisions around how much to push George and how much to let go. She wipes the back of her hand on her forehead and says to Kim, "I'll get him up in a bit, just as soon as I finish in here." Shirley knows that if George doesn't eat, he will continue to get weaker and weaker. She is often in the position of having to answer to people about how he's doing and how he's eating. It's exhausting and worrisome. Before she has to answer all the usual questions from Kim, they both hear her granddaughter yelling out back and calling for her mom. Kim heads out the back door to investigate.

By suppertime, the kitchen is full with George and Shirley's three children and their families. George is sitting in a captain's chair at the head of the table while the rest of the world moves around him. Chris and his teenage daughter, Jenny, are setting the table; the four younger grandchildren are playing a board game on the floor; Kim and her sister, Denise, are helping their mother put the boiled dinner on the table while the television is on in the background broadcasting the news. At least three conversations are going on at once; none of them involve George.

Shirley had dressed George in his red and blue flannel shirt and quilted vest. When she finally takes a seat, she notices how pale he looks. His eyes are dark and unfocused. Denise, who is an occupational therapist, sits next to him and helps him eat. She holds up the glass of milk and gives him a few sips to get his throat going. She flattens a carrot slice with a fork and feeds him a small amount. In between, she takes a few bites of her own dinner, and then resumes feeding her dad. The dinner conversation moves from talk of school to the increase in business at the farm, thanks to Halloween, and what the kids are going to dress up as. George doesn't say anything; he just nods from time to time when he's asked a question. Denise flattens a piece of potato, pours some milk and butter on it to make mashed potatoes, and feeds it slowly to her dad. She knows he could never handle a piece of the roast and would be chewing it forever, but he loves potatoes, especially mashed. After everyone has eaten and the kitchen is bustling again, Denise feeds her dad some of his favorite maple ice cream with his nighttime medicine.

The following morning, Shirley is in the kitchen creaming butter and sugar for brownies when she hears a woman call "Hello!" It must be the hospice nurse. Shirley heads out to the porch where George is sitting in his chair. "Hi, Charlene," Shirley says to her as she pulls up a chair and sits next to George. Shirley and Charlene start off by talking about the beautiful fall day and the busy farm stand. They try to involve George in the conversation, asking him about the farm, but his responses are short and vague.

"How are things going?" Charlene asks, looking back and forth between George and Shirley.

"Well, George's appetite has gone down quite a bit in the past week, and he is sleeping a lot more," Shirley begins. "He also seems more confused," she adds, lowering her voice to a whisper.

Charlene turns to George. "George, are you feeling sick to your stomach, or do you just not have much of an appetite?"

In response, George points his finger, implying the latter, "Not hungry."

"That's okay."

Shirley jumps in, "Some of my family, and George's family, keep pushing him to eat." She reaches over to hold George's hand. "I feel like he is slipping away," she says, her voice cracking as she reaches into her pants pocket, takes out a tissue, and wipes tears from her eyes.

Charlene reaches over and takes her hand now. "It's so hard—for everyone. Eating is such a family event. To feed people is to nurture them." She goes on to tell them that when people are really sick, they don't feel like eating. It's really hard for families to adjust to this, because everyone knows what happens when people don't eat. "It is normal, though, when people are in the final stage of life. It's also normal for families to feel sad and worried about it," Charlene says softly.

Shirley nods quickly and sits up straight.

"If you'd like, I can have our social worker, Pat, come out and visit with you and your family. You can talk about all these changes and what to expect in the weeks ahead."

Shirley looks over at George. He is dozing off again.

"We can give it a try," Shirley says tentatively.

"Shirley, we also have a really nice home health aide, Luz. She can come over three days a week to help bathe, dress, and walk with George, if you'd like. It might give you a bit of a break, at least a few times a week."

"Let me just run it by George," Shirley says, "but it sounds like it would help."

Over the next several weeks, George becomes weaker and eventually it becomes too much effort for him to get out of bed. He is now sleeping most of the day and night. His brother visits every few days, and the kids and grandkids are in and out most days. The refrigerator is full of food offered by friends, neighbors, and people from the church. George has regular visits from the minister and the hospice chaplain, Carole. George has an old Bible that he's had for years. The cover is worn and the pages are folded, but his favorite verses are bookmarked and Carole reads them to him every time she visits.

Shirley consistently tells Charlene that George seems very comfortable. The only time he winces is when he is turned. The nurses reinforce the importance of turning him over side to side regularly to keep his skin clean and to prevent bedsores.[1] Charlene encourages Shirley and the family to premedicate George with pain medicine a half an hour before turning him to make it easier for him to move.[2] George is only taking "sips and bites" of food now. Everyone now understands that it won't get better than this, and eventually, he won't take anything at all. They keep his mouth clean and fresh and put balm on his lips.

Over the course of the next two weeks, many questions and uncertainties arise. "Don't we have to turn off the pacemaker? Shouldn't he have some oxygen? What about an IV?" Charlene reassures them that these are questions that come up a lot; they should feel free to ask whatever questions they hear or think of. An implanted defibrillator is generally turned off, but not usually a pacemaker.[3] Oxygen isn't needed right now; he is breathing easily and doesn't seem to be short of breath. Intravenous fluids won't help at this point, and they might even make things worse.[4] It's better and more natural to not have too much extra fluid added. Charlene encourages them to call anytime they have questions or if they are worried about what's going on. She also tells them that they are taking wonderful care of George and encourages them to let hospice know how else they might be able to help.

A week later, Charlene and Pat make a late-afternoon visit together to see George and his family. The three children have been taking turns caring for George overnight so their mother can sleep. Sometimes their dad sleeps for three to four hours in a stretch, but other times, he is awake more often and seems restless. They turn him, clean him, and give him medicine that Charlene has prefilled. They are all bleary-eyed and worried about each other. George has not had anything to eat or drink in over a week.

Shirley and her children all gather in the kitchen with Charlene and Pat. They make some tea and coffee and put out snacks. When everyone has settled down at the table, Kim begins, her voice cracking, "I don't understand what he is waiting for!"

Pat calmly says, "He may or may not be waiting for anything, Kim. It's likely that he is in the final hours to days of life." She looks around at everyone at the table and continues, "I know you are all exhausted, but this won't go on for days. He will leave this world when he is ready and that won't be long."

Shirley eyes are drawn to the back window where the sun is starting to set; the reflection casts a warm orange glow in the room. She feels sad and weary. She hears Pat continue, but her voice sounds far away.

"Continue to keep him clean, calm, and comfortable. Reassure him, as you have, that he can go when he's ready; you will all be okay, and you'll look after your mom."

That night, it is Denise's turn to stay overnight and take care of her dad. She is awake with him until about 1 a.m., when he finally settles in and falls asleep. Denise, too, drifts off to sleep on the futon until 4 a.m., when she wakes up to go to the bathroom. She is startled by the silence. She jumps up to the bedside and discovers that her dad has died sometime in the last couple of hours. Denise places her hand on her mom's shoulder and whispers to her that he has died. Shirley and Denise go to George's side of the bed. Denise lays her head on her dad's shoulder while Shirley sits at his side, holds his hand, and weeps. They spend the next few moments in silence.

By the time Olga, the nurse on call, arrives for the pronouncement visit, the other children and family members have gathered. Everyone is drinking coffee, eating doughnuts, and talking about who they need to call, what they should bring to the funeral home, and when the services will likely occur. They are looking at pictures to include on a posterboard for the wake and telling stories about the past.

“Hey, Chris!” Kim calls over to her brother. “Here’s a picture of you and Dad on the tractor together. Dad always loved this picture.”

## REFLECTIONS ON GEORGE AND FAMILY

People often die when the threads that bind them to this world have let go. Saying goodbye to a spouse or parent can be tremendously sad. Some partners, like George and Shirley, have been together for more than fifty years. They have shared the world together for most of their lives. Families can help their loved ones be comfortable and at peace by giving bedside care, providing closure activities, and offering reassurances. Sometimes, however, it feels as though people are holding on. This is especially difficult when families are exhausted and stressed. Having patience and providing presence is important in the final days of someone’s life. Soon their body will no longer be there again. So often, it is their process and they will die when they are ready.

It can be very difficult to know how much to encourage people to eat and exercise when they are sick. This is one of the hardest experiences for families.[5] In the final months of life, it’s best to take cues from the person about how much they want. For example, sometimes people don’t feel like they have the energy to wash up, but once they do, they feel better. Offer but don’t insist. Try not to create the tense dynamic of constantly pushing someone to do more. It makes everyone feel badly.

People often engage in a life review in the final weeks and months of life. George was having lots of memories of his childhood. It's common for people who are dying to have recollections of their parents, or to relive experiences from when they were a child. George was sleeping a lot too, so he was probably experiencing lots of dreams. Sometimes, these end-of-life memories and/or visions provide peace and reconciliation from the past. Sometimes people find new meaning in their experiences and relationships.[6] Whatever the case, it helps to allow people to be wherever they need to be. If they're having distress during these experiences, family members and hospice can provide counseling and medication, if needed, as they go through this journey.

CHAPTER 15

# Soothing the Soul

Cindy's dad, Albert, always came home from business trips with a pewter spoon engraved with a new city on it for his little girl. She still has the entire collection. She smiles to herself, recalling how the three kids would plead with their mom to let them stay up until Dad got home. He would come through the door with a distinct aroma of wool and cedar, kiss Mom, put his hat on Paul's head, and scoop Joey into the air while Cindy wrapped her arms tightly around his leg. Her thoughts wander to these warm memories as she stares out the window and watches the trees sway in the wind.

Cindy and her brothers, Paul and Joe, are now taking turns caring for their dad since he was diagnosed with lung cancer four months ago. When their mom died three years ago, they created schedules, shopping lists, appointment reminders, and communication logs to help their dad stay at their family home. When he became weaker and needed more help with bathing and medical care, he moved in with Cindy, who is a nurse.

At this time, Albert is mostly staying in bed and sleeping off and on all day. He is only eating small amounts of custard and ice cream. Albert's favorite navy blue Air Force sweatshirt hangs loose on his shoulders. His frame, now pale and thin, is hard for Cindy to witness, as he was always so strong and full of life. Hospice is coming to Cindy's home to assist Albert and his family with his end-of-life care needs.

One afternoon, Cindy is in her study paying bills. Suddenly, her father screams. Cindy runs to his side, "Dad! Dad! What's the matter?" He's yelling in jumbled sentences and thrashing his arms around. It's as if he's having a bad dream and can't get out of it. Cindy fumbles in her pocket for her phone and calls her brother Joe and the hospice nurse.

The hospice nurse tells Cindy to give her dad a dose of haloperidol, a liquid medicine that is commonly given for agitation like this.[1] Cindy runs to the refrigerator to get the medicine, keeping an eye on her dad, who keeps grabbing and shaking the side rail of the hospital bed. Her fingers are shaking as she draws up the medicine in the eye dropper and gives him a dose by putting a few drops in the space between his bottom lip and teeth. "Dad, it's okay, it's Cindy." His eyes are open but unfocused, and he's gripping the side rail so tightly that his knuckles are white. Cindy tries to unpeel his fingers from the bed rail, but his grasp is firm. *How can he be so strong?*

After twenty harrowing minutes, her dad's forehead begins to relax slightly and his voice softens to a whisper. Joe rushes through the back door and comes to the other side of the bed. Cindy takes a deep sigh of relief. Although Albert has calmed down quite a bit, he still seems "unsettled." Cindy and Joe are rehashing the sequence of events when the hospice nurse, Charlene, arrives.

Cindy tells Charlene about how the day was going, what her dad ate, what medications he's had, and what they've done so far. After doing her assessment, Charlene recommends giving Albert some pain medication, cleaning him briefly, and turning him onto his favorite side with a pillow between his knees. All this seems to work as Albert's body begins to sink into the bed and his breathing becomes shallow and quiet.

Cindy, Joe, and Charlene move into the living room to talk about what's happening. Cindy sits on the couch as tears well up in her eyes. Joe sits on the edge of his dad's big, overstuffed recliner, hands held together tightly in his lap.

"You did the right thing; he's doing better now," Charlene tells them. "Unfortunately, restlessness and agitation are common at the end of life.[2] It can be very scary. Are you okay?"

Cindy takes a deep breath. "Yes, but I'm still reeling from this whole episode. It's hard to see him like this; I was afraid he was going to hurt himself."

"I know. It's incredible how strong people can be when they're so weak. It usually takes quick action, like you did, to de-escalate the situation. There are a number of things that we can do that will help, including arranging a respite stay for him, if you want."

Both Cindy and Joe speak of their insistence on caring for their dad until the end. "We don't want him to go to the hospital or a nursing home if it can be avoided. We've talked about it," Cindy says, looking over at Joe. "He wants to die here. We owe it to him, and besides, we promised our mother before she died that we would take care of Dad."

"Well, I totally support that, and I want to make sure that you're all okay, too," Charlene says as she grabs a booklet from her bag. "Our hospice put together this booklet; it is one of the most helpful things we give to families. It explains what commonly happens in the final stages of life." Charlene reviews sections of the booklet with them and then writes down instructions on how to give the medicines "around the clock" to prevent his agitation from starting up again.

Cindy tells Charlene and Joe that she's still worried about her dad's episode of agitation. "I was trying to figure out what he was saying. He kept mumbling about a train; he also kept repeating the word 'sky.' I wonder if he was having a bad dream."

After a few minutes, Charlene asks Cindy and Joe, "By any chance, is your dad a veteran?"

"Yes," Cindy says. "In fact, my Aunt Louise, his sister, told me that when he first came home from the service, he came down the long driveway of their home, went upstairs and took off his uniform, and never said another word about it."

"Well, that's not uncommon, especially for some veterans. It's hard to know, especially now, if he's having agitation because of any previous experiences. He could be encountering distress from visions of the war, things he witnessed, actions he may have taken, or fear of judgment. It's hard to know, but these things can weigh heavily on a person's soul."[3]

"I don't know," Joe muses. "He's never really said anything, except about the planes he flew and a few stories about some of his comrades."

Cindy agrees. "I've never heard him say that anything bad happened either. But he wasn't one to talk a lot about that anyway."

"Sometimes it helps for people to see their faith leader or our hospice chaplain. I know your dad is Catholic. I think it would be a good idea to ask a priest to come out and visit. He can offer prayers, reconciliation, and the Anointing of the Sick. It might help." Joe jumps up and offers to call their church and ask if a priest can come over as soon as possible.

Cindy tells Charlene that she is worried about future episodes of her dad's agitation. She retells the sequence of events, how it started, what he was yelling, and how he was acting. "It was so hard for me to see him like that," Cindy says as she moves a wad of tissues between her hands. "I wish I knew what was going on. I've never seen him like that."

"It sounds very difficult," Charlene offers. "It's hard to know, in these situations, what might be going on. We just try to keep people safe and offer care that we hope can bring someone some peace and comfort. I wonder if one of your brothers can stay with you overnight until we can be assured that your dad will stay calm."

"Probably, that's a good idea; I'll ask them."

"I'll also ask our social worker and chaplain to reach out to you. They have both helped many families with similar circumstances. I think it would help."

"Sure, I guess," Cindy says as she gets up to check on her dad.

Charlene packs up her supplies and reviews the instructions for medications and bedside care. She hugs them both and says, "Please call us for anything."

Later that afternoon, Charlene calls back to check on Albert. "It was like a magic wand!" Cindy says. "Father Dominic came over and blessed him and said prayers with Dad. Both of my brothers were here too; it was such a nice moment for us all. Now he's calm and looks like he's sleeping."

"Oh, thank goodness!" Charlene says, relieved. "I'm so glad he's better." She reviews with Cindy the medication plan again and the importance of skin and mouth care. She also encourages them to continue talking with him and offering him reassurances.

"Oh, we've been doing that. We told him that we love him and that he can go when he's ready; Mom is waiting for him."

"And how are you all holding up?"

"We're hanging in there."

All through the night and the following day, Albert rests calmly while Cindy, Paul, and Joe take turns caring for him. They know it won't be long, so they try to enjoy the time they have with him and with each other. They share stories about their dad. They're still miffed about how little they know about his time in the service. They wish they had talked with him more about it. Cindy tells them that after their dad dies, she plans to reach out to Aunt Louise and ask her about it. There's also a bundle of papers in a box at his house. "There'll be a lot to sort out, I'm sure," Cindy says as she exhales hard and shakes her head.

Later that afternoon, Charlene and Pat, the hospice social worker, make a visit together. They reinforce the medication plan and the bedside care. They're all relieved that Albert has remained calm. Pat offers additional help from a volunteer and home health aide. They decline, concluding that, "We're okay for now."

That night, sometime in the early morning hours, Albert died peacefully.

## REFLECTIONS ON ALBERT AND FAMILY

Agitation is a very challenging situation for families and hospice to deal with. When a dying person is confused, agitated, or unresponsive, it's not always clear what they're saying or what they might want. This can be very difficult. As Cindy experienced, it can feel dangerous and out of control. Loved ones struggle to interpret the situation. There is a condition called terminal restlessness or terminal delirium that can occur in the final weeks of someone's life. It is characterized by severe agitation and disorientation.[4] It's important for caregivers to keep themselves and their loved one from getting hurt. The hospice team can guide families in evaluating the environment and interpreting what might be going on. Together, care can be provided that addresses the physical, emotional, social, and spiritual realms that people face as they pass through the final stages of life.

Albert needed medication immediately to calm him down. Many people have mixed emotions about the use of medications at the end of—and throughout—life. Some families feel that hospice overuses medicine. Many people are afraid to give medications that are often prescribed at the end of life, especially haloperidol and morphine.[5] My experience is that, for many people and many diseases, going through the dying process "naturally," without medicine, often causes suffering. There are many non-medication actions that can be taken at the end of life that can help manage pain and agitation. However, medications are often critical, especially with terminal restlessness, to help someone who is dying stay safe and calm.

Many veterans do not talk about their service, sacrifice, and military experiences. They may have witnessed or participated in events that were deeply disturbing or impactful. Many veterans benefit from spiritual and emotional support in moving through these profound experiences.[6] Trauma-informed care is an approach to care that considers the pervasive nature of trauma and promotes environments of healing and recovery rather than practices that might inadvertently re-traumatize someone.[7] Prayers, rituals, and relics of one's faith can also be deeply comforting. Even when people have not been particularly religious in their adult life, many people find security and peace in past religious practices and blessings.[8] Spiritual counselors help people reflect on many religious and existential questions. All of these services can help people reconcile the events of their life and soothe their soul.

CHAPTER 16

# Bringing Dad Home to Die

Charlie has been through the mill and back. He's lying in a bed in the hospital, unresponsive and breathing deeply through his oxygen mask. He has a full head of gray hair, now moist and brushed away from his face, and a patchwork of bruises in various shades of red and purple up and down his arms. Charlie was admitted to the hospital a week ago with worsening heart and kidney failure. He spent several days in the intensive care unit where he underwent numerous tests and treatments in an attempt to stabilize his condition. Unfortunately, he kept getting worse and ended up on a breathing tube and attached to various monitors and IV lines. After talking with the hospital doctor, Charlie's daughter, Lauren, decided to take him off all the tubes and bring him home to die.

Lauren is sitting in a chair at the end of the bed, texting on her phone, when two people knock on the door. They introduce themselves as Charlene and Pat, the nurse and social worker from hospice. The hospital case manager called them to help coordinate Charlie's transfer home.

They gather around Charlie's bed. Lauren's long brown hair is pulled back in a ponytail and sunglasses rest on top of her head. She's still dressed in her black stretch pants, gray T-shirt, and sandals from this morning's yoga class. She tries to explain everything that's happened since her dad was admitted to the hospital, but it comes out like a detailed series of events that feel out of order. "I'm sorry, it's been crazy," she says as she rubs her eyes and blinks hard.

"I'm sorry your dad has been so sick," Pat says. "It sounds like he's gone through a lot."

Charlene reaches over and touches Charlie's shoulder. "We're going to help you get him transferred home and settled in." Charlene excuses herself to speak with the hospital nurse and doctor while Pat stays and hears Charlie's story from Lauren.

"My dad's had a lot of medical problems over the past two years. He's been in and out of the hospital at least three times in the past year. He hasn't been this sick; but the last time, he had to go to a rehab unit after the hospital. He hated it there. He kept asking to come home," Lauren says to Pat. "That's why I want to take him home; that's what he'd want." Lauren reports that she had a meeting with the doctor and decided to elect "comfort measures only" and signed a Do Not Resuscitate (DNR) form. Lauren takes a deep breath and then says, as she looks over at her father, "He's had a long, tough life."

Charlene speaks with the hospital doctor and goes over the details of the supplies and medicine that Charlie will need at home. She makes arrangements for a hospital bed, oxygen, and other supplies to be delivered to his home later that day. Charlene also coordinates the delivery of a morphine pump and reviews prescriptions with the doctor that will be faxed to the pharmacy near Charlie's home. She then goes back into Charlie's hospital room and relays all the plans to Lauren. Lauren tells them that her brother, Scott, and his wife are at the house now and can help receive all the supplies. She will pick up the prescriptions on her way there.

"Make sure he has the DNR form when he goes home in the ambulance," Charlene reminds her.

"Lauren, is your dad religious?" Pat asks. "Would you like us to arrange a visit by clergy or our hospice chaplain?"

"No, we're all set, thanks. His minister has come twice since he's been in the hospital. I'll give him a call later on when he gets home."

"Okay, then. We'll see you at the house," Charlene says as she packs up her belongings. "Lauren, we'll help keep your dad comfortable until he dies, and we'll take care of you and your family too."

Charlene arrives at Charlie's house late in the afternoon and parks on the street out front. The house is a small brick Cape Cod with a closed-up front door and a porch entrance on the right, between the house and the garage. The driveway, and the yard to the right of the driveway, is full with cars, trucks, and several motorcycles. It's starting to get dark out, but with the porch light she can see a small gathering of men outside. As she's collecting her supplies from the trunk, she notices an American flag and a POW/MIA (prisoner of war / missing in action) flag on a pole to the left of the garage. As she walks toward the porch, she sees that most of the men are wearing leather vests covered with patches and embroidered with "American Legion Riders." They're huddled around talking while some are drinking beer and smoking cigarettes. Charlene greets them, introduces herself, and says, "I'm sorry about Charlie."

One of his friends opens the door for Charlene as she goes into the porch. After knocking on the door, she enters the kitchen and follows the path through the kitchen and around to the left, where the hospital bed is set up in the living room up against the wall. All the furniture has been pushed to the other side of the room along the window. Scott is sitting in a recliner going through a stack of papers while Lauren is at the end of the bed, spreading a blanket out over her dad.

"Oh, hi!" Lauren says when she sees Charlene. "We made it."

Charlene smiles as she walks over to the side of the bed. "Welcome home, Charlie," she says. Charlie is lying slightly upright in the hospital bed. His eyes are closed and he's unresponsive. "His breathing seems a bit more labored than when I saw him at the hospital, so I'm going to start the morphine pump." Lauren passes her the bag that was delivered with the medicine and all the supplies. Charlene inserts a small needle in Charlie's belly and attaches the medicine. She presses the bolus dose button on the machine and explains to Lauren and Scott that this will raise his breathing comfort level.

Charlene does her usual assessment, all the while teaching Scott and Lauren about the medications, when to give them, how to turn him, what to look for, and when to call. She also offers additional help from the hospice team, which they readily accept: "We'll take all the help we can get."

Once Charlie is settled and breathing more comfortably, Charlene, Scott, and Lauren talk about what to expect. Charlene hands them a booklet that explains what signs and symptoms are common in the final hours and days of someone's life. "I'm kinda familiar with a lot of this cuz I used to work as a nurse's aide in a nursing home," Lauren tells them. "I know it's not the same when it's your own family."

"No, it isn't. For sure. But since you're familiar with a lot of this, it will be easier," Charlene reassures her.

Scott glances up at his father and then quickly flips through the booklet.

Charlene points to the pages that talk about the final signs that people often go through. “It’s common for people to have changes in their skin color, sometimes pale or gray, and even bluish areas on their legs and hands,” Charlene explains. “This is normal. Sometimes people have restlessness, congestion, or a fever.[1] You have medicine here that will help with any of that, if it happens.” Charlene picks up each medicine bottle and explains what it’s for and how to give it. She passes each one to Lauren, who reads the label and then puts them on the table. “If anything comes up, or your dad doesn’t seem comfortable, you should call us,” Charlene tells them.

“Now that we’ve gone over the medical stuff, tell me a little bit about your dad.”

Scott and Lauren look at each other and then Lauren begins, “Well, he and my mom got divorced when we were six and eight, or something like that. She lives in Florida now. He drank a lot back then, but he’s been sober now for years. There was a period of time when we didn’t see him that much,” Lauren says. Scott adds that they are all on good terms now. He sees his dad about every week or two, usually to watch a hockey or basketball game on TV. Lauren nods in agreement. “I talk with him on the phone about every day or two and see him at least once a week. He’s been sick a lot lately, though, so I’ve seen him more, to take him to appointments and stuff.”

Just then, they hear the porch door close and men talking in the kitchen. “Those guys have been great,” Lauren says, pointing toward the kitchen. “Dad has been riding with his Legion buddies for years. They’ve been so helpful, especially this past year.” When Charlene asks what branch of the service he was in, Scott points to a black cap on the table with “US Army Veteran” and the Army seal printed on the front. “He loves that hat,” Lauren says as she reaches over and puts the hat on her dad's head. Charlene smiles as she packs up her bag, hugs both kids, and rubs Charlie's cheek. She reminds them to call if they have any questions or they don't think he's comfortable.

Lauren is sleeping on the couch when she wakes to the sound of her father's breathing and the oxygen tank swishing. She looks at her phone and the bright light says 3:05 a.m. She flings the fleece blanket off and jumps up to her dad's bedside, holding on to the bed rail. His face looks red and wet and his breathing sounds like he has phlegm in his throat. She reaches her right hand up and places it on his forehead. *He feels awfully hot*, she thinks as she wonders what she did with that thermometer. She remembers what the nurse had said, that she should call if anything comes up, so she reaches back to the couch for her phone and calls the number for hospice.

After Lauren tells the operator what's going on, the hospice nurse on call, Marie, calls her back. She gives her instructions on what to do now, and then tells her that she will be there shortly. Lauren looks for the bed controls and presses the "up" button and her father sits up a bit more. She then fixes his oxygen tube so the prongs are squarely in his nose. She pushes the button on the morphine pump, as she was instructed to do, and hears the "zing" sound that indicates that a dose was given. She then goes into the kitchen, opens the refrigerator, looks at the labels of the emergency medicine, and grabs the one that says "for secretions." She shakes the bottle and opens the cap to see an eye dropper attached to the cap. She carefully pulls down her father's lower lip and squeezes out two drops of the liquid into his mouth. With each step, she talks to her dad, tells him what she's doing and that she hopes it will help him rest better. Lauren then goes into the bathroom and looks around the sink and closet for the forehead thermometer. Not finding it, she goes over and sits on the toilet. She bends over, puts her face in her hands, and then realizes that she still has the same clothes on that she's had on all day.

Marie arrives and comes up along the bedside next to Lauren. Lauren tells her what she's done since they talked. When Marie completes her assessment, she tells Lauren that her dad has a fever and congestion, not just in his throat but in his lungs. His breathing rate is also elevated and he's having periods of not breathing at all for ten to fifteen seconds. Marie explains to Lauren that this is called "apnea" and it's common.[2] Giving doses of both morphine and lorazepam will help keep his breathing calm, but the congestion is a bit harder to manage.[3] The medication to treat secretions might help some, but laying him flat and way over onto his side will help move the phlegm away from his throat.[4] "It's so hard to listen to," Lauren says. "It sounds like he's drowning."

"I know. I wish I could make it go away," Marie says, "but turning him onto his side will help." They move the bed away from the wall slightly as Lauren squeezes into the space between the bed and the wall and lowers the side rail. She follows Marie's lead, and they turn Charlie onto his side and put a pillow between his knees and a towel under his cheek. Lauren goes back into the refrigerator and brings Marie the medicine labeled "fever." Marie administers an acetaminophen suppository to Charlie, then they both push the bed back in place and cover him with just a light sheet.

While Marie washes up and packs her bag, Lauren taps out a message to her brother on her phone. Marie and Lauren hug goodbye and then Lauren says, "He looks and sounds so much better now."

Lauren goes into the kitchen, drinks a glass of water, unlocks the back door, and then sits back on the couch. She feels both hyperalert and overwhelmingly fatigued at the same time. She lies back down, checks her phone, and eventually dozes off. She is awoken by the sound of her brother opening the cabinet in the kitchen. When he comes into the living room, she updates him on what's been going on. Lauren then reshuffles, hugs her pillow, and pulls the blanket up over her shoulder. Scott is sitting in the chair near the bed looking at his phone as she drifts back off to sleep.

"Lauren! Lauren!" Scott says quickly as he stands up to get a better look at his father's face. "His breathing has changed," he tells Lauren as she stands up at the bedside, still holding onto the blanket. They both look at their dad as he takes a long breath in and a short, quick breath out. Lauren bends over the side rail, kisses him on the forehead, and says "We love you, Dad." Scott rubs his dad's thigh and says "Love you, Dad." After only two more breaths, his chest doesn't rise again. Lauren and Scott look at each other, eyes wide, and then back at their dad. "You can finally rest now, Dad."

## REFLECTIONS ON CHARLIE AND FAMILY

Although many people want to die at home, it isn't possible or practical for everyone. Sometimes, the situation is just too demanding and overwhelming. Lauren was familiar with bedside care and she knew her dad wouldn't live for very long. It takes a lot of communication and coordination between family members, hospice, and health care facilities to transfer someone who is dying back home. It can be incredibly satisfying for family to have their loved one home. Even when people who are dying aren't fully awake, they seem to sense the familiar smells, sounds, and "feel" of home.

Throat mucus in a dying person is very difficult for families to experience.[5] I really do wish there was a magic wand to get rid of it. It mostly happens when someone is very close to death and they're so weak that they can't clear their throat. It's hard to know how much people who are dying experience it, since they are generally unresponsive when it occurs. Some people refer to it as the "death rattle," but I prefer to use words like "throat secretions" or "throat mucus," which sound softer. There is medicine that can help, but depending on the circumstances, it might not make it go away. Suctioning isn't generally recommended either. Putting a tube in someone's mouth near their throat could stimulate their gag reflux and cause them more distress. Positioning people on their side can help as much as anything.[6] Managing this symptom, like others, helps everyone have a more peaceful end-of-life experience.

CHAPTER 17

# Saying Goodbye

Terri goes upstairs to check on her sister. Brenda is lying still and quiet under a pale lavender sheet, her long black hair spilling over the pillow. Her body seems so small in the double bed. Brenda is in the final days of her short, thirty-one-year life.

Hospice is called in at the very end to help care for Brenda, who is experiencing restlessness. Brenda is dying from complications of AIDS (acquired immunodeficiency syndrome). It isn't clear how long Brenda has had the disease, how she got it, or what she has gone through. The focus now is to bring her symptoms under control so she is more at peace.

Charlene reviews the referral paperwork from the doctor's office and begins the drive over to Brenda's house. She reflects on her long hospice nursing career. She hasn't cared for many people with AIDS; thankfully there is treatment now that can manage the disease. During the onset of AIDS in the early 1980s, she remembers a young Puerto Rican man with AIDS who lived in an inpatient unit. Sadly, he was isolated and stigmatized. The only one who was able to connect with him was another Spanish-speaking man from the kitchen, who came up and read to him regularly from the Bible. Another man she cared for with AIDS became incredibly thin before he died. He had long hair and a beard. Charlene couldn't help thinking that, with his skeletal body, he looked just like Jesus Christ. His family had so much shame about his disease that they were insistent that his death certificate not say that he'd died from AIDS. Fatal diseases that are contagious always seem to cause so much fear and sorrow. Yet for people who are dying and their families, what matters in the end is that their loved ones are comfortable, peaceful, and well cared for until they die.

Charlene is greeted at the door by Brenda's two sisters, Elaine and Terri. She is welcomed into the kitchen, where they both talk rapidly, back and forth, to give Charlene a report on what's been going on. Brenda has been restless and agitated, off and on, for the past twenty-four hours. "Nothing seems to help for very long," Elaine says as they usher Charlene upstairs to Brenda's bedroom.

Charlene gently lifts the sheet from Brenda's body and touches the fragile skin on her back. She notices a small butterfly tattoo on her scapula or "wing bone," which is now prominently elevated from her back. Brenda seems mildly restless. Her legs are drawn up in a fetal position and her arms are moving up and down. She is unresponsive and unable to communicate what she might need or what might be bothering her. Charlene is struck by how thin she is. Brenda's face is sunken and every bone is visible in her petite frame. She barely weighs seventy pounds.

Charlene grabs supplies from her bag and proceeds to listen to Brenda's lungs, checks her temperature, and begins to uncover what might be causing her to have these severe periods of agitation. She doesn't have a fever and her lungs are clear. Her skin color is very pale, in stark contrast to her long black hair. She's so young.

Elaine and Terri are on either side of Brenda's bed. The resemblance between them is striking. They both have light brown hair, hazel eyes, and a short, slightly heavy frame. The oldest, Elaine, speaks first. "I set up this medicine schedule," she says, picking up a notebook from the bedside table. With the pen, she points to her notes about the fentanyl patch for pain, when she put it on, and when it's due to be changed. She moves on to list the next medicine, lorazepam. "I give this when she's restless and moving around a lot. It doesn't always help, though."

Terri jumps in. "This morning was bad—that's why I called the doctor. She was yelling and thrashing around in the bed. Her eyes were open but she didn't seem to see us. Nothing we said or did calmed her down."

"We gave her some liquid pain medicine and lorazepam and she finally started to relax," Elaine explains. "I don't know if the medicine helped or if she finally conked out from being up all night, but she's been like this since."

Charlene asks several questions about Brenda's symptoms, medications, and the timing of these outbursts. She wonders whether her agitation might be more related to emotional or spiritual distress than from physical symptoms. Charlene makes a call to the hospice social worker and spiritual counselor, who both agree to visit. Carole, the hospice spiritual counselor, is able to come over right away.

Charlene talks with Elaine and Terri about common symptoms that can occur at the end of someone's life. Restlessness and agitation can be extremely frightening and exhausting. It can be hard to pinpoint the cause. Charlene reassures them that there are many steps that can be taken to help this situation. She takes some haloperidol and lorazepam from the emergency kit and sets up a schedule of these medications. "When people experience severe restlessness and agitation, these medicines can often help calm them down."[1]

Just then, they hear a knock on the door and head downstairs to greet Carole.

Carole is one of those people whose eyes shine bright with compassion. She deals with many spiritual and metaphysical concerns. She talks with people about vast end-of-life questions, such as: What do I believe? What happens after I die? Have I been a good person in this life? Why has God forsaken me? and Will I ever be forgiven? She has helped many families face this end-of-life journey. Charlene and Carole sit across from Elaine and Terri and begin to learn Brenda's story.

"She's had a tough life," Terri begins. "She's our middle sister, smart as a whip and funny as hell. Unfortunately, she got involved with drugs. Soon, she started hanging around with a rough crowd and began shooting heroin."

"She's been in and out of detox and rehab a few times, and was even in jail once," Elaine adds. "That was terrible for her and her daughter, Karlie. Karlie is Brenda's seven-year-old daughter. She is the spitting image of Brenda, with dark hair and sharp eyes. She is in the second grade but is reading at a fourth-grade level. Karlie is a huge animal lover. She has so many stuffed animals, you can't even see her bed!" Charlene and Carole talk with Brenda's sisters about how they and Karlie are coping with Brenda's illness and impending death. They learn that Karlie has a lot of support from them, her cousins, and a counselor at school. Brenda was never particularly religious, so they decline outside spiritual support. Elaine and Terri say they are managing. "It's sad, but we'll get through it. If she stays peaceful, we can handle it. We've been doing okay so far."

Carole asks Brenda's sisters, "Who will take care of Karlie after Brenda dies?" They both agree; Terri is the logical choice as she is Brenda's health care proxy, and besides, she has two children who are also in elementary school. They never had any explicit conversation with Brenda about this, but Terri and Elaine "figured that Brenda knew the plan."

Carole asks Elaine and Terri for permission to speak with Brenda along with her sisters. They encircle her bed. Brenda's eyes are closed, her body is calm, and her breathing is very shallow. Carole talks with them about hope and forgiveness. "You never really lose hope—it's just that what you hope for often changes over time. Sometimes it's hoping to live longer, sometimes it's to have a peaceful death, and other times, it's hoping that everyone will be okay."

Elaine and Terri tell Brenda that they love her. They reassure her that Karlie will be loved and cared for by both sisters and will live with Terri and her family. "We will make sure that Karlie never forgets you, Brenda." They cry, laugh, and have silent moments together.

Carole encourages Elaine and Terri to have Karlie say goodbye to her mom when she gets home. She also encourages Karlie to make a memory book to remember her mom by. She can write down stories, draw pictures, or use stickers to express her feelings. "These memories may comfort her in the years to come." Carole reminds them that the hospice social worker will be visiting later today and will help them with that. As Carole is getting ready to leave, she tells them that she is also the hospice bereavement counselor and will be keeping in touch with them for at least a year after Brenda dies.

During the next two days, Karlie and her aunts have many sweet conversations with Brenda. They hug her, sing songs to her, and say their final goodbyes.

## REFLECTIONS ON BRENDA AND FAMILY

Many families ask hospice how they can help children deal with death. Providing simple, honest, and age-appropriate information is important. Listening carefully to children, guiding any misconceptions, and providing security and love all help.[2] Counseling and group support can also encourage them to share their feelings with others.[3] Children often hold dear photos, videos, and scrapbooks of their parents or loved ones, especially if they are young when the death occurs.[4] These firsthand words and drawings become windows to the experience long after someone dies. They help create treasured memories for years to come.

Taking care of another human being who is at the end of life is a precious gift. Whether it's your spouse, parent, sibling, child, or another family member or friend, the experience is incredibly meaningful. Be gentle with yourself and others. Take it all one day at a time. Your love and care are a blessing.

CONCLUSION

# Final Words

I am tremendously grateful to the many families and coworkers who have helped me develop my understanding and passion for quality end-of-life care. Families have allowed me to walk into their lives and share their homes, relationships, and emotions. They have taught me much about life, death, grief, and love. Our journey together has also given me an outlook on life that allows me to see every person as valuable and every moment as precious.

I hope this book helps you understand how important it is for all adults to choose a health care surrogate or proxy. This is someone you assign to make health care decisions for you if you are unable to make them yourself. People with a serious illness should also talk with their health care providers about which medical procedures would be advisable for them in emergency situations. Having these "advanced directive" discussions and filling out the appropriate medical-legal forms can help avoid a lot of chaos and regrets during and after an emergency.[1]

Unfortunately, I have witnessed overtreatment and burdensome care in many people who are sick. The care they have received has not made them better, nor have they had a positive health care experience. It's not easy to know when to forgo additional tests, treatments, and hospitalizations. It requires guidance by medical professionals who understand the stages of illness and the benefits and burdens of various medical treatments.[2] More is not always better. Sometimes it's better for people with an advanced illness to stay home and be surrounded by the people and pets who love them. They can move around in familiar surroundings, eat home-cooked food, and sleep in their own beds. It is often a safer and more satisfying experience than acute medical care—if that care cannot make someone better.

I am both amazed and saddened by the number of sick and elderly people who are transferred between home, hospitals, and nursing homes in the final two years of their lives. It seems particularly sad to me when these people have dementia and memory loss. All these transitions have inherent risks for people who are seriously ill and frail. This is when palliative care providers can help families decide what to do.[3] They help clarify what's necessary versus potentially burdensome. They focus on what's most important to the person and their family.

Another important step to minimize suffering in people who are sick or dying is to manage symptoms that come up. Many people hold deep personal, cultural, and religious beliefs about pain and suffering. They have the right to uphold these beliefs and to make medical decisions in accordance with these beliefs. However, there is a tremendous amount of misinformation and lack of knowledge about symptoms and how to manage them. Symptom management is a health care specialty. Research continues to advance our understanding of symptoms and effective ways to manage them. More education is needed, not just about medications but also about holistic approaches and integrative therapies for managing symptoms. In many cases, the relief of pain, difficulty breathing, restlessness, and other symptoms is what allows people to have a peaceful dying process and death.[4]

Many of the stories in this book have revealed family experiences with palliative care and hospice. I hope this has provided you with a better understanding of both programs and how they work. My experience is that both palliative care and hospice provide holistic and compassionate health care and the clinicians connect with people, first and foremost, on a human-to-human level.

For many families, care of a loved one at the end of life exists within the context of their culture and religion. Beliefs, values, relics, and traditions are often central to the experience of dying and death. As a clinician, learning about such a wide variety of cultural experiences has been tremendously enriching. My direct exposure to a fuller spectrum of cultural experiences has been limited, however, by the area where I have practiced.

Hospice and palliative care programs face the challenge of being accessible to many families of color. Despite continued growth in these programs, racial disparities continue to exist.[5] Decisions about whether to seek acute medical care rather than hospice care are deeply personal. These discussions rely on a trusting relationship with medical staff who recognize and appreciate the values and beliefs of each family. It also underscores the importance of having medical providers who represent diverse backgrounds and share the same culture and language of the people they care for.

I have included additional information on end-of-life care in the bibliography. Families can contact local hospice agencies directly to request information. Medicare rates the quality of hospice programs, just as it does for hospitals and nursing homes.[6] This reference is also included in the bibliography.

Palliative care access is currently more limited. Most palliative care providers work in hospitals, and their services are limited to people who are hospitalized. However, more and more, palliative care services are becoming available on an outpatient basis. The standardization of services and the payment for palliative care is evolving.

Dying and death affect all of us. It's very scary and personal, but we shouldn't be afraid to look ahead and learn more about it. Perhaps if people talked more about death, we would have a better understanding of what happens when people die. I believe we would also be more aware of the choices available and more comfortable with the whole process. This would create opportunities for better end-of-life care.

I hope you have enjoyed reading about these families caring for loved ones who are dying. I also hope their stories have helped clarify the dying process and what can make the experience a little easier. If you find yourself in the same position as many of these families, I hope this book shines a light on what can be done during this time and guides you through the difficult but meaningful journey ahead.

# ACKNOWLEDGMENTS

This book is about families and the care they provide to their loved ones. I am deeply indebted to my own family, who have provided me with endless love and support throughout the writing of this book. At every step along the way, my husband, John Lasek, has been there to support my end-of-life work and writing. My children, Matthew and Annie Lasek, have given me immeasurable love and encouragement. The wit and kindness of my family always lifts my spirits. My siblings are like lifelong friends. They remind me of the importance of staying grounded, being devoted, and maintaining a sense of humor.

I am grateful to the early readers of my manuscript: Alicia O. M. Ross, MD, Olga Ehrlich, RN, Diana Federman, Jim Palermo, Lindsay Whiting, Annie Lasek, and John Lasek. Their guidance gave me the encouragement and motivation I needed to keep writing.

A thank-you to the professionals who provided invaluable feedback on my manuscript: book coach Lindsay Whiting and editors Celia Jeffries, Laura Carney, Jean Zimmer, and Ellie Barton. In addition, I am blessed to have wonderful friends and family with expertise in end-of-life care and writing. Thank you to Olga Ehrlich, RN, Jeff Zesiger, MD, Alicia O. M. Ross, MD, Karen Aroian, RN, and my sister, Patty Whitney, MD, for your expert consultation and advice. I have also received valuable guidance from authors: Maureen Stanton, Jennifer Rogala, Emily Everett, Maureen Callahan Smith, and Lewis Cohen, MD. Thank you all for your encouragement and support.

I have had the good fortune to be represented by Joan Parker, of the Parker Literary Agency. Joan's professional and practical advice has helped me immensely. I would like to thank my editor, Suzanne Staszak-Silva, and the team at Johns Hopkins University Press: Robert Brown, Nicole Wayland, Kris Lykke, and Kait Howard. Thank you for recognizing the importance of educating families about end-of-life care through storytelling. Your faith in me and in *When a Loved One Is Dying* will help many readers learn valuable lessons about caring for family members who are seriously ill or dying.

It takes a team to care for people at the end of life—so does writing a book. Thank you to all the patients and families, literary professionals, colleagues, and friends and family who have championed this book and helped bring it into the world.

# NOTES

Chapter 1. I Can't Believe This Is Happening

1. Coyne et al., "American Society for Pain Management," 328.
2. National Cancer Institute, "Cancer Pain."
3. End-of-Life Nursing Education Consortium, "Final Hours."
4. National Institute on Aging, "Providing Care and Comfort."
5. Mendoza, "Facing Death Together."

Chapter 2. Does Palliative Care Mean That Mom Is Dying?

1. Center to Advance Palliative Care, "America's Readiness."
2. Get Palliative Care, "Palliative Care."
3. Hospice Foundation of America, "What Is Hospice?"
4. Caring Info, "Types of Care."
5. Family Caregiver Alliance, "Pathways to Effective Communication."
6. Michel et al., "Key Aspects of Psychosocial Needs," 8.

Chapter 3. Good Days and Bad Days

1. Ibitoye et al., "Frailty," 147.
2. Hospice and Palliative Nurses Association, "Patient Nearing the End of Life."
3. Cohen et al., "Hope," 1344.
4. ACP Decisions, "Benefits of Advance Care Planning."
5. Prepare for Your Care, "PREPARE."

6. The Conversation Project, "Your Guide."
7. Byock, *Consider the Conversation*, 34:44–36:46.

### Chapter 4. When Is Active Treatment No Longer Worth It?

1. Alzheimer's Association, "Stages of Alzheimer's."
2. Sclan and Reisberg, "Functional Assessment Staging," 58–59.
3. Alzheimer's Disease Research Center, "Identifying Swallowing Difficulties."
4. Alzheimer's Foundation of America, "Eating and Dementia."
5. Alzheimer's Association, "Stages of Alzheimer's."
6. Centers for Medicare and Medicaid Services, "Hospice Determining Terminal Status."
7. Caring Info, "Types of Care."

### Chapter 5. How Long Does Mom Have to Live?

1. Metheny, "Preventing Aspiration."
2. Palliative Care Network of Wisconsin, "Fast Fact #3: Syndrome of Imminent Death."
3. Karnes, *Gone from My Sight*, 13–14.
4. End-of-Life Nursing Education Consortium, "Final Hours."
5. Hospice and Palliative Nurses Association, "Patient Nearing the End of Life."
6. Chu et al., "Prognostication," 306.
7. National Institute on Aging, "Making Decisions."

### Chapter 6. From Discord to Harmony

1. Hospice and Palliative Nurses Association, "Medically Administered Nutrition."
2. Lindskog et al., "Fluid Therapy," 4.

3. Warden et al., "PAINAD," 12.
4. Herr et al., "Pain Assessment," 563–64.
5. Stuart et al., "Role of Families," 1147.
6. Alzheimer's Association, "Memory Loss and Confusion."

## Chapter 7. The Family Circle at the End of Life

1. Hui et al., "Management of Dyspnea," 1390–91.
2. Bovero et al., "Loss of Personal Autonomy," 182.
3. National Consensus Project, *Domain 6: Cultural.*

## Chapter 8. Dealing with the Crisis of Pain

1. Karnes, *Gone from My Sight*, 13–14.
2. Paice et al., Use of Opioids," 920.
3. Henson et al., "Palliative Care," 906.
4. Hoff et al., "Hospice Satisfaction," 698.
5. El-Jawahri et al., "Psychological Distress," 491.
6. Caring Info, "Types of Care."

## Chapter 9. Morphine Doesn't Kill People, Diseases Do

1. Harsanyi et al., "Stigma Surrounding Opioid Use," 5841.
2. Kwekkeboom et al., "Revisiting Patient-Related Barriers," 1845.
3. Hui et al., "Management of Dyspnea," 1391.
4. Campbell et al., "Treatment of Dyspnea," 409.
5. Hui et al., "Management of Dyspnea," 1391.
6. National Institute on Aging, "Providing Care and Comfort."
7. End-of-Life Nursing Education Consortium, "Final Hours."
8. Hospice and Palliative Nurses Association, "Patient Nearing the End of Life."

## Chapter 10. Managing Anxiety and Restlessness

1. World Health Organization, *WHO Guidelines*, 37; Hospice and Palliative Nurses Association, "Patient Nearing the End of Life."
2. Rogers et al., "ONS Guidelines," 676.
3. Paice et al., "Use of Opioids," 916.
4. World Health Organization, *WHO Guidelines*, 33.
5. National Center for Complementary and Integrative Health, "Anxiety."
6. National Consensus Project, *Domain 3: Psychological*.

## Chapter 11. I Just Can't Do This Anymore

1. Campbell et al., "Treatment of Dyspnea," 409.
2. Oliver, "Mysteries, Yes," 62. Reprinted by the permission of The Charlotte Sheedy Literary Agency as agent for the author. Copyright © 2009, 2017 by Mary Oliver with permission of Bill Reichblum
3. Skantharajah et al., "Grief and Bereavement Experiences," 246.
4. Glass et al., "Concordance of End-of-Life Care," 5; Cypher and Axman, "Determinants of Location of Death," 1401.

## Chapter 12. Nothing Left Unsaid

1. End-of-Life Nursing Education Consortium, "Final Hours."
2. Pakenham and Martin, "Psychosocial," 748.
3. Masterson et al., "Beyond the Bucket List," 2574.

## Chapter 13. Keeping Things Normal

1. National Hospice and Palliative Care Organization, *Hospice Medication*.

2. American Nurses Association, *Code of Ethics*, 9.
3. National Consensus Project, *Domain 8: Ethical and Legal*.

### Chapter 14. The Agony of Waiting for Dad to Die

1. Vickery et al., "Pressure Injury Prevention," 574.
2. Coyne et al., "American Society for Pain Management," 328.
3. Stoevelaar et al., "Advance Care Planning," 912; American Heart Association, "Planning for Advanced Heart Failure."
4. Lindskog et al., "Fluid Therapy," 4.
5. Palliative Care Network of Wisconsin, "Fast Fact #470: Counseling Adult Patients."
6. Rabitti et al., "Hospice Patients' End-of-Life Dreams," 109.

### Chapter 15. Soothing the Soul

1. Ellsworth et al., "Risk Factors and Antipsychotic Usage," 205.
2. Watt et al., "Incidence and Prevalence of Delirium," 871.
3. US Department of Veterans Affairs, "PTSD: National Center."
4. Soroka et al., "Terminal Delirium in Hospice," 27.
5. Gerber et al., "Barriers to Adequate Pain and Symptom Relief," 6; Gerlach et al., "Benzodiazepine and Antipsychotic Prescribing," 1301.
6. Pless Kaiser et al, "Factors Associated with Distress," 108.
7. Duchowny et al., "Prevalence of Lifetime Trauma," 131.
8. Balboni et al., "Spirituality in Serious Illness," 194.

Chapter 16. Bringing Dad Home to Die

1. Hospice and Palliative Nurses Association, "Patient Nearing the End of Life."
2. Hospice Foundation of America, "When Death Is Near."
3. Hui et al., "Management of Dyspnea," 1389.
4. Hospice and Palliative Nurses Association, "Terminal Secretions."
5. Oliver et al., "Sights and Sounds of Respiratory Changes," 193.
6. Palliative Care Network of Wisconsin, "Fast Fact #109: Death Rattle and Oral Secretions."

Chapter 17. Saying Goodbye

1. Hui et al., "Pharmacologic Management of End-of-Life Delirium," 9.
2. Hoppe et al., "When a Parent Dies," 6.
3. National Alliance for Children's Grief, "Find a Support Center."
4. Schonfeld, et al., "Supporting the Grieving Child," 4.

Conclusion

1. ACP Decisions, "Benefits of Advance Care Planning."
2. Qureshi et al., "End-of-Life Burdensome Transitions," 7.
3. Get Palliative Care, "Palliative Care."
4. Mather et al., "Symptom Management Experience," 513.
5. Parajuli et al., "Barriers to Palliative and Hospice Care," 12; National Alliance for Care at Home, "NHPCO Facts and Figures 2024."
6. Centers for Medicare and Medicaid Services, "Find and Compare: Hospice."

# BIBLIOGRAPHY

ACP Decisions. "19 Evidence-Based Benefits of Advance Care Planning." Last modified October 15, 2020. https://www.acpdecisions.org/19-evidence-based-benefits-of-advance-care-planning/.

Alzheimer's Association. "Memory Loss and Confusion." Accessed January 15, 2025. https://www.alz.org/help-support/caregiving/stages-behaviors/memory-loss-confusion.

Alzheimer's Association. "Stages of Alzheimer's." Accessed January 15, 2025. https://www.alz.org/alzheimers-dementia/stages.

Alzheimer's Disease Research Center. "Identifying Swallowing Difficulties: The Role of the Caregiver." Last modified March 15, 2021. https://www.adrc.wisc.edu/news/identifying-swallowing-difficulties-role-caregiver.

Alzheimer's Foundation of America. "Eating and Dementia." Accessed January 15, 2025. https://alzfdn.org/eating-tips/.

American Heart Association. "Planning for Advanced Heart Failure." Last modified July 13, 2023. https://www.heart.org/en/health-topics/heart-failure/living-with-heart-failure-and-managing-advanced-hf/planning-ahead-advanced-heart-failure#.

American Nurses Association (ANA). *Code of Ethics for Nurses with Interpretive Statements.* American Nurses Association, 2015.

Balboni, Tracy A., Tyler J. VanderWeele, Stephanie D. Doan-Soares, Katelyn N. G. Long, Betty R. Ferrell, George Fitchett, Harold G. Koenig, Paul A. Bain, Christina Puchalski,

Karen E. Steinhauser, et al. "Spirituality in Serious Illness and Health." *JAMA: Journal of the American Medical Association* 328, no. 2 (July 2022): 184–97. https://doi.org/10.1001/jama.2022.11086.

Bovero, Andrea, Rossana Botto, Elena Mellano, Francesco Gottardo, Paola Berchialla, Sara Carletto, and Giuliano C. Geminiani. "Loss of Personal Autonomy and Dignity-Related Distress in End-of-Life Cancer Patients." *American Journal of Hospice and Palliative Medicine* 41, no. 2 (February 2024): 179–86. https://doi.org/10.1177/10499091231166373.

Byock, Ira, interviewee. *Consider the Conversation: A Documentary on a Taboo Subject.* Produced by Michael Bernhagen and Terry Kaldhusdal, A Burning Hay Wagon Production, 2011, 34:44–36:46.

Campbell, Margaret, DorAnne Donesky, Alexandra Sarkozy, and Lynn Reinke. "Treatment of Dyspnea in Advanced Disease and at the End of Life." *Journal of Hospice and Palliative Nursing* 23, no. 5 (October 2021): 406–20. https://doi.org/10.1097/NJH.0000000000000766.

Caring Info, a program of the National Alliance for Care at Home. "Types of Care." Accessed January 15, 2025. https://www.caringinfo.org/types-of-care/.

Center to Advance Palliative Care. "America's Readiness to Meet the Needs of People with Serious Illness: 2024 Serious Illness Scorecard, August 2024. https://scorecard.capc.org/.

Centers for Medicare and Medicaid Services. "Find and Compare Providers Near You: Hospice." Accessed February 1, 2025. https://www.medicare.gov/care-compare/?providerType=Hospice.

Centers for Medicare and Medicaid Services. "Local Coverage Determination (LCD): Hospice Determining Terminal Status." Last modified June 27, 2024. https://www.cms.gov/medicare-coverage-database/view/lcd.aspx?LCDId=34538.

Chu, Christina, Nicola White, and Patrick Stone. "Prognostication in Palliative Care." *Clinical Medicine* 19, no. 4 (July 2019): 306–10. https://doi.org/10.7861/clinmedicine.19-4-306.

Cohen, Michael G., Andrew D. Althouse, Robert M. Arnold, Hailey A. Bulls, Douglas B. White, Edward Chu, Margaret Q. Rosenzweig, Kenneth J. Smith, K., and Yael Schenker. "Hope and Advance Care Planning in Advanced Cancer: Is There a Relationship?" *Cancer* 128, no. 6 (March 2022): 1339–45. https://doi.org/10.1002/cncr.34034.

Conversation Project, an initiative of the Institute for Healthcare Improvement. "Your Guide to Choosing a Health Care Proxy." 2021. https://theconversationproject.org/wp-content/uploads/2020/12/ChooseAProxyGuide.pdf.

Coyne, Patrick, Sarah Lowry, Carol Mulvenon, and Judith A. Paice. "American Society for Pain Management Nursing and Hospice and Palliative Nurses Association Position Statement: Pain Management at the End of Life." *Pain Management Nursing* 25, no. 4 (August 2024): 327–29. https://doi.org/10.1016/j.pmn.2024.03.020.

Cypher, Mackenzie, and Linnea M. Axman. "Determinants of Location of Death: A Secondary Analysis Utilizing Multinomial Logistic Regression." *American Journal of Hospice and Palliative Medicine* 39, no. 12 (March 2022): 1397–1402. https://doi.org/10.1177/10499091221077883.

Duchowny, Kate A., Alexander K. Smith, Irena Cenzer, Chelsea Brown, Grace Noppert, Kristine Yaffe, Amy L. Byers, Carla

Perissinotto, and Ashwin A. Kotwal. "The Prevalence of Lifetime Trauma and Association with Physical and Psychosocial Health Among Adults at the End of Life." *Journal of the American Geriatrics Society* 73, no. 1 (October 2024): 123–35. https://doi.org/10.1111/jgs.19209.

El-Jawahri, Areej, Joseph A. Greer, Elyse R. Park, Vicki A. Jackson, Mihir Kamdar, Simone P. Rinaldi, Emily R. Gallagher, Annemarie D. Jagielo, Carlisle E. W. Topping, Madeleine Elyze, et al. "Psychological Distress in Bereaved Caregivers of Patients with Advanced Cancer." *Journal of Pain and Symptom Management* 61, no. 3 (March 2021): 488–94. https://doi.org/10.1016/j.jpainsymman.2020.08.028.

Ellsworth, Emily M., Kevin J. Bacigalupo, Kavita R. Palla, Seema S. Limaye, Margaret J. Walkosz, Sandra T. Szczecinski, and Katie J. Suda. "Risk Factors and Antipsychotic Usage Patterns Associated with Terminal Delirium in a Veteran Long-Term Care Hospice Population." *Federal Practitioner: For the Health Care Professionals of the VA, DoD, and PHS* 38, no. 5 (May 2021): 202–8. https://doi.org/10.12788/fp.0131.

End-of-Life Nursing Education Consortium (ELNEC). "Final Hours Supplemental Materials." Last modified 2020. https://www.aacnnursing.org/Portals/42/ELNEC/PDF/ELNEC-Final-Hours-of-Life-Supplemental.pdf.

Family Caregiver Alliance. "Pathways to Effective Communication for Health Care Providers and Caregivers." Last modified 2021. https://www.caregiver.org/resource/pathways-effective-communication-healthcare-providers-and-caregivers/.

Gerber, Katrin, Lindy Willmott, Ben White, Patsy Yates, Geoffrey Mitchell, David C. Currow, and Donella Piper. "Barriers to Adequate Pain and Symptom Relief at the End of Life: A Qualitative Study Capturing Nurses' Perspectives."

*Collegian* 29, no. 1 (2022): 1–8. https://doi.org/10.1016/j.colegn.2021.02.008.

Gerlach, Lauren B., Molly Turnwald, Kristin Geczi, Thomas O'Neil, Daphne Watkins, Julie P. W. Bynum, and Donovan T. Maust. "Factors Associated with Benzodiazepine and Antipsychotic Prescribing in Hospice: A Qualitative Study of Hospice Prescribers." *Journal of the American Medical Directors Association* 24, no. 9 (September 2023): 1297–1302. https://doi.org/10.1016/j.jamda.2023.04.007.

Get Palliative Care, provided by Center to Advance Palliative Care. "Palliative Care: What You Should Know," 2019. https://getpalliativecare.org/wpcontent/uploads/2021/01/GPC_WhatYouShouldKnowHandout_2019.pdf.

Glass, David P., Susan E. Wang, Paul M. Minardi, and Michael H. Kanter. "Concordance of End-of-Life Care with End-of-Life Wishes in an Integrated Health Care System." *Jama Network Open* 4, no. 4 (April 2021): 1–12, e213053. https://doi.org/10.1001/jamanetworkopen.2021.3053.

Harsanyi, Hannah, Colleen Cuthbert, and Fiona Schulte. "The Stigma Surrounding Opioid Use as a Barrier to Cancer-Pain Management: An Overview of Experiences with Fear, Shame, and Poorly Controlled Pain in the Context of Advanced Cancer." *Current Oncology* 30, no. 6 (June 2023): 5835–48. https://doi.org/10.3390/curroncol30060437.

Henson, Lesley A., Matthew Maddocks, Catherine Evans, Martin Davidson, Stephanie Hicks, and Irene J. Higginson. "Palliative Care and the Management of Common Distressing Symptoms in Advanced Cancer: Pain, Breathlessness, Nausea and Vomiting, and Fatigue." *Journal of Clinical Oncology* 38, no. 9 (March 2020): 905–14. https://doi.org/10.1200/JCO.19.00470.

Herr, Keela, Alison R. Anderson, Caroline Arbour, Patrick J. Coyne, Elizabeth Ely, Céline Gélinas, and Renee C. B. Manworren. "Pain Assessment in the Patient Unable to Self-Report: Clinical Practice Recommendations in Support of the ASPMN 2024 Position Statement." *Pain Management Nursing* 25, no. 6 (December 2024): 551–68. https://doi.org/10.1016/j.pmn.2024.09.010.

Hoff, Timothy, Kathryn Trovato, and Aliya Kitsakos. "Hospice Satisfaction Among Patients, Family, and Caregivers: A Systematic Review of the Literature." *American Journal of Hospice and Palliative Medicine* 41, no. 6 (June 2024): 691–705. https://doi.org/10.1177/10499091231190778.

Hoppe, Rebecca, Marcia A. Winter, Chelsea D. Williams, and Irwin Sandler. "When a Parent Dies: A Scoping Review of Protective and Risk Processes for Childhood Bereavement." *Death Studies* (April 2024): 1–11. https://doi.org/10.1080/07481187.2024.2340729.

Hospice and Palliative Nurses Association (HPNA). "HPNA Nursing Resource Guide: Care of the Patient Nearing the End of Life. Accessed January 15, 2025. https://www.advancingexpertcare.org/wp-content/uploads/2023/08/6_NRG_End-Of-Life.pdf.

Hospice and Palliative Nurses Association (HPNA). "HPNA Nursing Resource Guide: Terminal Secretions. Accessed February 1, 2025. https://www.advancingexpertcare.org/wp-content/uploads/2023/08/NRG-Terminal-Secretions-Final-2023-1.pdf.

Hospice and Palliative Nurses Association (HPNA). "Position Statement: Medically Administered Nutrition and Hydration." Last modified January 2020. https://www.advancingexpertcare.org/wpcontent/uploads/2023/05/HPNA

_Position_Statement_MedicallyAdministeredNutrition.Hydration.pdf.

Hospice Foundation of America. "What Is Hospice?" Last modified September 24, 2024. https://hospicefoundation.org/what-is-hospice/.

Hospice Foundation of America. "When Death Is Near: Signs and Symptoms." Last modified September 24, 2024. https://hospicefoundation.org/when-death-is-near-signs-and-symptoms/.

Hui, David, Kari Bohlke, Ting Bao, Toby Campbell, Patrick Coyne, David C. Currow, Arjun Gupta, Aliza L. Leiser, Masanori Mori, Stefano Nava, et al. "Management of Dyspnea in Advanced Cancer: ASCO Guideline." *Journal of Clinical Oncology* 39, no. 12 (April 2021): 1389–1411. https://doi.org/10.1200/JCO.20.03465.

Hui, David, S. Y. Cheng, and Carlos E. Paiva. "Pharmacologic Management of End-of-Life Delirium: Translating Evidence into Practice." *Cancers* 16, no. 11 (May 2024): 2045, 1–13. https://doi.org/10.3390/cancers16112045.

Ibitoye, Sarah E., Sadie Rawlinson, Andrew Cavanagh, Victoria Phillips, and David J. H. Shipway. "Frailty Status Predicts Futility of Cardiopulmonary Resuscitation in Older Adults." *Age and Ageing* 50, no. 1 (January 2021): 147–52. https://doi.org/10.1093/ageing/afaa104.

Karnes, Barbara. *Gone from My Sight: The Dying Experience*. Rev. ed. BK Books, 2024.

Kwekkeboom, Kristine, Ronald C. Serlin, Sandra E. Ward, Thomas W. LeBlanc, Adeboye Ogunseitan, and James Cleary. "Revisiting Patient-Related Barriers to Cancer Pain Management in the Context of the US Opioid Crisis." *Pain* 162, no. 6 (June 2021):1840–47. https://doi.org/10.1097/j.pain.0000000000002173.

Lindskog, Magnus, Hanna Mogensen, Björn Tavelin, Johanna Eknert, Staffan Lundström, and Peter Strang. "Fluid Therapy Is Associated with Lower Care Quality and Higher Symptom Burden During Last Days of Life of Patients with Cancer—A Population-Based Register Study." *BMC Palliative Care* 23, no. 178 (July 2024): 1–8. https://doi.org/10.1186/s12904-024-01504-5.

Masterson, Melissa P., Elizabeth Slivjak, Greta Jankauskaite, William Breitbart, Hayley Pessin, Elizabeth Schofield, Jason Holland, and Wendy G. Lichtenthal. "Beyond the Bucket List: Unfinished and Business Among Advanced Cancer Patients." *Psycho-Oncology* 27, no. 11 (2018): 2573–80. https://doi.org/10.1002/pon.4821.

Mather, Harriet, Hannah Kleijwegt, Evan Bollens-Lund, Amy S. Kelley, and Katherine A. Ornstein. "Symptom Management Experience of End-of-Life Family Caregivers: A Population-Based Study." *Journal of Pain and Symptom Management* 64, no. 6 (December 2022): 513–20. https://doi.org/10.1016/j.jpainsymman.2022.07.017.

Mendoza, Marilyn A. "Facing Death Together at the Bedside: What to Do at the Deathbed." *Psychology Today*, January 14, 2018. https://www.psychologytoday.com/us/blog/understanding-grief/201801/facing-death-together-at-the-bedside.

Metheny, Norma A. "Preventing Aspiration in Older Adults with Dysphagia." Hartford Institute for Geriatric Nursing, ConsultGeri: Try This: Series, Issue #20 of General Assessment Series. Accessed January 15, 2025. https://hign.org/consultgeri/try-this-series/preventing-aspiration-older-adults-dysphagia.

Michel, Cathrin, Hannah Seipp, Kathrin Kuss, Michaela Hach, Andrea Kussin, Jorge Riera-Knorrenschild, J., and Stefan

Bösner. "Key Aspects of Psychosocial Needs in Palliative Care: A Qualitative Analysis within the Setting of a Palliative Care Unit in Comparison with Specialised Palliative Home Care." *BMC Palliative Care* 22, no. 100 (July 2023): 1–11. https://doi.org/10.1186/s12904-023-01227-z.

National Alliance for Care at Home. "NHPCO (National Hospice and Palliative Care Organization) Facts and Figures 2024 Edition." September 2024. https://allianceforcareathome.org/facts-and-figures-report-2024-edition/.

National Alliance for Children's Grief. "Find a Support Center or Camp Near You." Accessed February 3, 2025. https://nacg.org/find-support/.

National Cancer Institute. "Cancer Pain (PDQ)–Patient Version." Last modified September 17, 2024. https://www.cancer.gov/about-cancer/treatment/side-effects/pain/pain-pdq#_8.

National Center for Complementary and Integrative Health (NCCIH). "Anxiety and Complementary Health Approaches." Accessed January 27, 2025. https://www.nccih.nih.gov/health/anxiety-and-complementary-health-approaches.

National Consensus Project for Quality Palliative Care. *Clinical Practice Guidelines for Quality Palliative Care: Domain 3: Psychological and Psychiatric Aspects of Care.* 4th ed. National Coalition for Hospice and Palliative Care, 2018. https://www.nationalcoalitionhpc.org/ncp.

National Consensus Project for Quality Palliative Care. *Clinical Practice Guidelines for Quality Palliative Care: Domain 6: Cultural Aspects of Care*. 4th ed. National Coalition for Hospice and Palliative Care, 2018. https://www.nationalcoalitionhpc.org/ncp.

National Consensus Project for Quality Palliative Care. *Clinical Practice Guidelines for Quality Palliative Care: Domain 8:*

*Ethical and Legal Aspects of Care.* 4th ed. National Coalition for Hospice and Palliative Care, 2018. https://www.nationalcoalitionhpc.org/ncp.

National Hospice and Palliative Care Organization (NHPCO). *The NHPCO Hospice Medication Deprescribing Toolkit.* Version 1, November 2020. https://www.nhpco.org/wp-content/uploads/NHPCO_Deprescribing_Toolkit.pdf.

National Institute on Aging. "Making Decisions for Someone at the End of Life: Cultural Considerations at the End of Life." Last modified November 17, 2022. https://www.nia.nih.gov/health/end-life/making-decisions-someone-end-life#cultural-considerations-at-the-end-of-life.

National Institute on Aging. "Providing Care and Comfort at the End of Life." Last modified November 17, 2022. https://www.nia.nih.gov/health/end-life/providing-care-and-comfort-end-life.

Oliver, Debra Parker, Masako Mayahara, Allison Donehower, Jacquelyn J. Benson, Daniel Paget, Keisha White Makinde, Justin Daniels, and Patrick White. "Sights and Sounds of Respiratory Changes During Hospice Death Vigils: Hospice Caregivers Experience." *Journal of Pain and Symptom Management* 69, no. 2 (February 1, 2025): 190–95. https://doi.org/10.1016/j.jpainsymman.2024.10.035.

Oliver, Mary. "Mysteries, Yes." In *Evidence: Poems*. Beacon Press, 2009. Line in chapter 11 reprinted with permission of the Charlotte Sheedy Literary Agency as agent for the author. Copyright 2009, 2017 by Mary Oliver with permission of Bill Reichblum.

Paice, Judith A., Kari Bohlke, Debra Barton, David S. Craig, Areej El-Jawahri, Dawn L. Hershman, Lynn R. Kong, Geana P. Kurita, Thomas W. LeBlanc, Sebastiano Mercadante, et al. "Use of Opioids for Adults with Pain from

Cancer or Cancer Treatment: ASCO Guideline." *Journal of Clinical Oncology* 41, no. 4 (February 2023): 914–30. https://doi.org/10.1200/JCO.22.02198.

Pakenham, Kenneth, and Christina L. Martin. "Psychosocial Palliative Care: Patients' Preferred Intervention Medium, Target Domains, and Well-Being Priorities." *Palliative and Supportive Care* 22, no. 4 (August 2024): 742–50. https://doi.org/10.1017/S1478951522001535.

Palliative Care Network of Wisconsin. "Fast Fact #3: Syndrome of Imminent Death." Last modified April 1, 2024, by David E. Weissman. https://www.mypcnow.org/fast-fact/syndrome-of-imminent-death/.

Palliative Care Network of Wisconsin. "Fast Fact #109: Death Rattle and Oral Secretions." Last modified February 11, 2019, by Kathleen Bickel, Lava Kareem, Trinh Bui, and Robert M. Arnold. https://www.mypcnow.org/fast-fact/death-rattle-and-oral-secretions/.

Palliative Care Network of Wisconsin. "Fast Fact #470: Counseling Adult Patients and Caregivers on Nutrition During the Dying Process." Last modified October 5, 2023, by Kimberly Tyler, Chad Glisch, Juan Pagan-Ferrer, and April Zehm. https://www.mypcnow.org/fast-fact/counseling-adult-patients-and-caregivers-on-nutrition-during-the-dying-process/.

Parajuli, Jyotsana, Aluem Tark, Ying-Ling Jao, and Judith Hupcey. "Barriers to Palliative and Hospice Care Utilization in Older Adults with Cancer: A Systematic Review." *Journal of Geriatric Oncology* 11, no. 1 (January 2020): 8–16. https://doi.org/10.1016/j.jgo.2019.09.017.

Pless Kaiser, Anica, Jennifer Moye, Lola Baird, Zachary Sager, and Melissa Wachterman. "Factors Associated with Distress Related to Posttraumatic Stress Disorder at the End of Life

Among US Veterans." *Journal of Pain and Symptom Management* 66, no. 2 (August 2023): 102–15. https://doi.org/10.1016/j.jpainsymman.2023.04.011.

Prepare for Your Care. "PREPARE." Licensed by the Regents of the University of California. Accessed January 15, 2025. https://prepareforyourcare.org/en/welcome.

Qureshi, Danial, Nicholas Grubic, Colleen J. Maxwell, Shirley H. Bush, Genevieve Casey, Sarina R. Isenberg, Peter Tanuseputro, and Colleen Webber. "Association of Disease Trajectory and Place of Care with End-of-Life Burdensome Transitions: A Retrospective Cohort Study." *Journal of the American Medical Directors Association* 25, no. 11 (November 2024): 1–14, 105229. https://doi.org/10.1016/j.jamda.2024.105229.

Rabitti, Elisa, Silvio Cavuto, Matías Eduardo Díaz Crescitelli, Maria Chiara Bassi, and Luca Ghirotto. "Hospice Patients' End-of-Life Dreams and Visions: A Systematic Review of Qualitative Studies." *American Journal of Hospice and Palliative Medicine* 41, no. 1 (January 2024): 99–112. https://doi.org/10.1177/10499091231163571.

Rogers, Barbara, Pamela K. Ginex, Allison Anbari, Brian J. Hanson, Kristine B. LeFebvre, Rachael Lopez, Deborah M. Thorpe, Brenda Wolles, Kerri A. Moriarty, Christine Maloney, et al. "ONS Guidelines for Opioid-Induced and Non-Opioid-Related Cancer Constipation. *Oncology Nursing Forum* 47, no. 6 (November 2020): 671–91. https://doi.org/10.1188/20.ONF.671-691.

Schonfeld, David J., Thomas Demaria, Arwa Nasir, and Sairam Kumar. "Supporting the Grieving Child and Family: Clinical Report." *Pediatrics* 154, no. 1 (July 2024): 1–13. https://doi.org/10.1542/peds.2024-067212.

Sclan, Steven G., and Barry Reisberg. "Functional Assessment Staging (FAST) in Alzheimer's Disease: Reliability, Validity and Ordinality." *International Psychogeriatrics* 4, no. 3 (April 1992): 55–69. https://doi.org/10.1017/S1041610292001157.

Skantharajah, Neerjah, Carol Barrie, Sharon Baxter, M. Carolina Borja, Anica Butters, Deborah Dudgeon, Ayeshah Haque, Iqra Mahmood, Mehrnoush Mirhosseini, Raza M. Mirza, et al. "The Grief and Bereavement Experiences of Informal Caregivers: A Scoping Review of the North American Literature." *Journal of Palliative Care* 37, no. 2 (April 2022): 242–58. https://doi.org/10.1177/08258597211052269.

Soroka, Jacek T., Krista J. Fling, Jennifer M. Heibel, Gregory R. Kutcher, and Sarah J. Ward. "Terminal Delirium in Hospice: The Experiences and Perspectives of Caregivers Providing Care to Terminally Ill Patients in Home Settings." *American Journal of Hospice and Palliative Medicine* 39, no. 1 (January 2022): 27–33. https://doi.org/10.1177/10499091211000729.

Stoevelaar, Rik, Arianne Stoppelenburg, Rozemarijn L. van Bruchem-Visser, Anne Geert van Driel, Dominic A. M. J. Theuns, Martine E. Lokker, Rohit E. Bhagwandien, Agnes van der Heide, and Judith A. C. Rietjens. "Advance Care Planning and End-of-Life Care in Patients with an Implantable Cardioverter Defibrillator: The Perspective of Relatives." *Palliative Medicine* 35, no. 5 (May 2021): 904–15. https://doi.org/10.1177/02692163211001288.

Stuart, Laura Braithwaite, Catrin Hedd Jones, and Gill Windle. "A Qualitative Systematic Review of the Role of Families in Supporting Communication in People with Dementia." *International Journal of Language and Communication Disorders* 57, no. 5 (September 2022): 1130–53. https://doi.org/10.1111/1460-6984.12738.

US Department of Veterans Affairs. "PTSD: National Center for PTSD: Moral Injury." Last modified August 2, 2024, by

Sonya B. Norman and Shira Maguen. https://www.ptsd.va.gov/professional/treat/cooccurring/moral_injury.asp.

Vickery, Jessica, Lauren Compton, Jackie Allard, Terri Beeson, Joycelyn Howard, and Joyce Pittman. "Pressure Injury Prevention and Wound Management for the Patient Who Is Actively Dying: Evidence-Based Recommendations to Guide Care." *Journal of Wound, Ostomy and Continence Nursing* 47 (2020): 569–75. https://doi.org/10.1097/WON.0000000000000702.

Warden, Victoria, Ann C. Hurley, and Ladislav Volicer. "Development and Psychometric Evaluation of the Pain Assessment in Advanced Dementia (PAINAD) Scale. *Journal of the American Medical Directors Association* 4, no. 1 (January–February 2003): 9–15. https://doi.org/10.1097/01.JAM.0000043422.31640.F7.

Watt, Christine L., Franco Momoli, Mohammed T. Ansari, Lindsey Sikora, Shirley H. Bush, Annmarie Hosie, Monisha Kabir, Erin Rosenberg, Salmaan Kanji, and Peter G. Lawlor. "The Incidence and Prevalence of Delirium Across Palliative Care Settings: A Systematic Review." *Palliative Medicine* 33, no. 8 (September 2019): 865–77. https://doi.org/10.1177/0269216319854944.

World Health Organization. *WHO Guidelines for the Pharmacological and Radiotherapeutic Management of Cancer Pain in Adults and Adolescents*. World Health Organization, 2018. https://www.who.int/publications/i/item/9789241550390.

# INDEX

## ABOUT THE AUTHOR

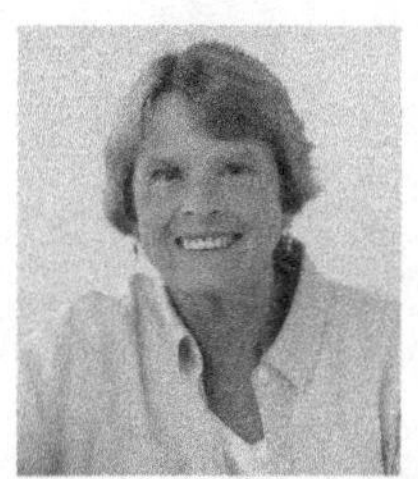
Courtney Saulnier Doherty Photography

**Maureen Groden** is passionate about helping families experience a peaceful end-of-life journey. She uses storytelling to help readers understand what happens when people are dying and how to care for them.

Maureen has been a hospice nurse leader and educator for several decades. She obtained her undergraduate and graduate degrees in nursing. She holds certification as a hospice and palliative care registered nurse. Maureen has conducted numerous presentations on end-of-life care in the professional arena as well as in the community.

*When a Loved One Is Dying: Conversations About Care, Connection, and Coping* illuminates a deeply personal but often phenomenal experience.